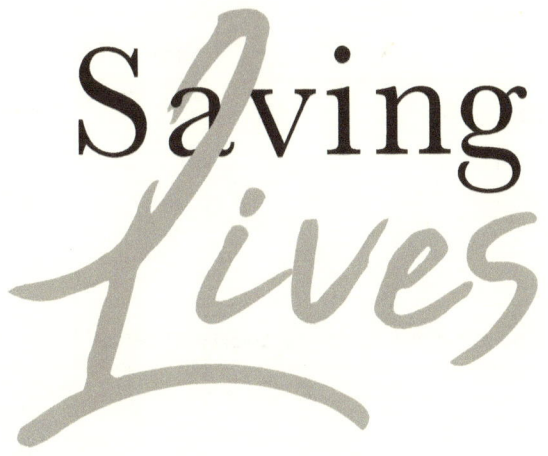

Saving Lives

Possibly Yours Or Someone You Love

Stephen Marks, Ph.D.

with Denise Rogers

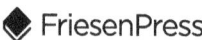

FriesenPress

Suite 300 - 990 Fort St
Victoria, BC, V8V 3K2
Canada

www.friesenpress.com

Copyright © 2019 by Stephen Marks and Associates Limited
First Edition — 2019

All rights reserved.

ISBN
978-1-5255-4694-5 (Hardcover)
978-1-5255-4695-2 (Paperback)
978-1-5255-4696-9 (eBook)

1. BIOGRAPHY & AUTOBIOGRAPHY, MEDICAL

Distributed to the trade by The Ingram Book Company

Medical Disclaimer
The information contained in this book is intended to provide helpful and informative material on the subject addressed. It s not intended to offer or to serve as a replacement for professional medical advice. Any use of the information in this book is at the reader's discretion. The authors and publisher disclaim any and all liability arising directly and indirectly from the use or application of any information contained in this book.

Table of Contents

to Denise

My partner in health, in love and life
and to all the Health Professionals who care for us.

Foreword

My initial vision for this section was to have everyone I encountered on my "adventure" contribute to the foreword to capture the experience from their perspective and in their own words. Unfortunately, this objective fell far short of my initial target. First of all, I tried unsuccessfully to get all of the "angels" who appeared to assist Denise and me to contribute, which none of them did, with one notable exception, Dr. Emily Claspell whom we have known for many years.

The second group I intended to enlist were all the medical professionals in Hawaii that I encountered on this journey and again this task proved to be as challenging as the former one to achieve. It turned out that none of the doctors in the two hospitals I visited ultimately participated. However, Dr. Ben Azman did agree. He was the first doctor I saw and he thankfully launched me in the correct direction.

When I returned home, I had much better success since most of the people I asked to contribute gladly agreed.

My second intention was to write the foreword as close to the events as possible but as my efforts to collect "contributions" took much more time than I anticipated, I realized that there might be advantages in waiting a while to see how the story unfolded. As time passed and my efforts to gather "contributions" proved to be ongoing, it began to appear that writing the complete book after a five-year span did have some benefits.

Well it's been ten years, and I can report with confidence on what has happened.

The contributions to the foreword are listed in chronological order for the Hawaii portion of the story, beginning with Dr. Azman.

The contributions from people back home are placed into three groups: my nephews and a longtime friend and financial advisor; my doctors; and finally, two of my close professional associates and dear friends who also personally share this health adventure with me.

What follows are their comments:

Hawaii

Dr. Ben Azman
As a patient, Stephen Marks is unique in his efforts not only to understand his medical condition but also to educate and help others in preventing coronary artery disease. While he describes his experiences in illuminating detail, Denise Rogers gives us a poignant glimpse of the events as viewed by the spouse.

Ben K. Azman, M.D.
Medical Director
Urgent Care West Maui

Dr. Emily Claspell
It all began with a phone call. I will never forget the sound of Denise's voice, as she told me that Steve was flown by air ambulance from Maui to Oahu, and was expected to have major bypass surgery. She sounded so sad and exhausted. My mind was a whirl, as I had just spent time with Steve and Denise a few days before. And, although I thought Steve looked tired and seemed to be operating slower than

usual, I attributed his condition to one of fatigue, as he had just finished presenting at an international conference held on the Island of Hawaii.

As I read Steve and Denise's book, *Saving Lives: Possibly Yours Or Someone You Love*, the memories of that particular time came flooding back to me, as well as the intense emotions that I felt, as I read through the timeline and the detailed accounting of the events that took place. I was impressed that both Steve and Denise shared their stories and the impact of how these early events in the time line transformed their lives, even through today.

As Steve and Denise waited for the insurance issues to be sorted out before Steve's operation, I was frightened for Steve, and wondered if I would ever see my friend again. I was angry with the insurance hassles and reassured myself that Steve was a strong man, and he would be able to get through this challenge OK. I did not know at the time, that Steve welcomed that impasse to reflect on his life, and used that time to prepare himself mentally and emotionally for the surgery. I stayed in touch with Denise. I could tell that this experience was draining and how difficult it was to cope with all the logistics of moving their things out of their condo on Maui, and then settling on Oahu, where she could be close to Steve, and focus on her own self-care. I believe the book captures the essence of what individuals, couples, families and friends experience when there is a medical emergency. The events show the uncertainty of how the "not knowing" plays on our fears and anxieties, when we desperately want to focus on hope and reassurance.

"Saving Lives" does not skimp on the consequences of ignoring physical red flags that are signals that not all is as well as it should be. Both men and women are invested in keeping up the image that heart disease is not a possibility or a potential threat to their lives. This is especially true if the perception of yourself is that you are a strong and healthy being, and that you are able to stave off the symptoms when they emerge through denial or positive thinking (my body will heal itself). Why change your diet, take medication or examine your lifestyle, when you have always been able to do what you have wanted? Acknowledging symptoms is a function of weakness rather than strength in our society.

Steve's story is a result of holding on to some of these perceptions, and he is the first to admit that this kind of thinking got him into trouble. He shared an anecdote with me after he came out of surgery, where a fellow patient who had a similar operation was visiting with his family. They showed up with the typical "plate lunch" that is famous in Hawaii. These plates are comprised of a large helping of meat, usually deep fried, two scoops of rice, and salad (not green salad). The salad is usually macaroni salad or a combination of macaroni and potato salad (no veggies) made with gobs of mayonnaise. So after a multiple bypass operation, the thinking that all is now well in the kingdom, seems to be a reason to continue making unhealthy choices. I can only think of how helpful "Saving Lives" would have been to this patient and family, in making better food choices, and still expressing love and support by sharing something healthy and life affirming.

Both Steve and Denise are individuals who focus on service, so it was no surprise to me that they wanted to share their experiences to help others. The assessment of "Risk" at the beginning of the book, and the interventions toward the end of the book to improve overall cardiac health, serves as a template for raising consciousness and making proactive choices. Both Steve and Denise can attest to the challenges of these choices as described in the events during the months and years after the surgery. They both serve as excellent examples as to the vigilance it takes on both of their parts to support these changes. Some people who read this book may be overwhelmed by all of the good suggestions.

With this group, I would view the book and its action points as a starting place. Perhaps taking on one or two action points at a time, and integrating these into your life is a good first step, before adding on more.

I am grateful that this "awful" experience, turned into a life saver for Steve. I am looking forward to many more years of enjoying our friendship and spending quality time when we get together in Hawaii. *Mahalo*, Steve and Denise for your gift of "Saving Lives".

Emily Claspell, ED.D.
Kamuela, Hawaii

Home (Vancouver and Burnaby)

Nick Marks

My Uncle Steve's little adventure in Hawaii just happened to coincide with my move from the UK to Vancouver. I had the pleasure of being Steve's driver and assistant for a few weeks while I was job hunting, and therefore had just a bit of free time on my hands. I was glad to be able to lend a hand as Steve was on the path to recovery. Major heart surgery is obviously not for the faint of heart (no pun intended), and I could see that it had taken quite a bit out of Steve (I can now happily report that he is back to full health). I have to admit that I was impressed by Steve's food regime after his 'event'. I guess lots of people would view the heart surgery as a bit of a clean slate and a chance to carry on past eating/consumption habits (I probably thought this before Steve's surgery). But Steve, who has always had an interest in healthy food choices, continued, and even stepped up his pursuit of a heart healthy diet and food regime. I will freely admit that I have become more conscious of my own food choices after seeing what Steve went through – and I hope this will serve me well as I get older. As a final note, I'd like to report that I have been a guinea pig for a few of my uncle's recipes, and I can report that his alternative desserts work quite well and are rather tasty (I've gone back for seconds so that tells you all you need to know).

Nick Marks BA. Management Studies, MSc. Real Estate
Vice President, Real Estate Finance
Anthem Properties Group Ltd.

Jon Marks

It was a big shock for our whole family when we heard the news that my uncle needed to undergo urgent heart bypass surgery. For as long as I can remember, Stephen led a healthy lifestyle, watching what he ate, keeping a healthy weight, and regularly exercising.

I believe that these healthy habits enabled Stephen to make a strong recovery. I admire Stephen for writing this book and sharing his story to help and educate others based on his experience.

Jon Marks BSc. CPA, CA
Finance Manager
Whistler Community Services Society

Brian Sung
"Live Long & Prosper"

Like the logical and intrepid "Spock" on his lifelong voyage of discovery, Stephen's approach to life is measured and well considered. Having family history, Stephen instinctively knew that to lead a long life one must manage all the risks – physically, mentally and emotionally.

Stephen has always taken very good care of his physical body through diet, exercise, and lifestyle.

Knowing that "stress kills", it was logical to Stephen that one must also manage emotional and mental stress. A large portion of mental and emotional stress is concern over what would happen if financial income is adversely affected due to sickness and/or injury.

What would happen financially if you don't die, remain alive, but are severely incapacitated?

Critically Illness insurance resonated with Steve, which, as circumstances dictated, would later have a direct and beneficial effect on his life.

Critical Illness insurance reduced his mental and emotional stress! Reduced stress added to his general level of holistic and physical health. Along with his other lifestyle choices, which contributed to his overall level of health, Steve was able to overcome his "heart" event on Maui.

"Saving Lives" is an exciting and insightful chapter of the "ship's log" of the journey of Stephen's "heart".

Brian Sung, B. Comm., MBA, CA

Dr. Monte Glanzberg

I am flattered by Steve's request to contribute to the foreword of his book "Saving Lives". It is particularly rewarding that both his recovery from coronary artery bypass surgery and ongoing health have been excellent. This personal story, complemented by insights from his partner Denise, reveal an intimate look at the diagnosis and treatment of coronary artery disease from a patient's perspective. The preventative advice and suggestions are thoughtful, and hopefully will motivate others to intervene with meaningful and appropriate changes in lifestyle.

Monte M. Glanzberg, B.Sc., M.D., CCFP
Family Medicine

Dr. Saul Isserow

It is an honor to both pen a foreword for Stephen's book and to be involved in Stephen's care as he journeys through his life with coronary artery disease.

Stephen's journey, albeit a profoundly personal one, is shared with his readers in the hope that they too will develop insight into their cardiovascular risk. It is not only what we physicians can do about it, but what they can do about it themselves. This is paramount to their well-being and the partnership between concerned and dedicated health professionals and the individual is what determines, to a large extent, success or failure.

In Stephen's case, his commitment and dedication to managing his cardiovascular risks as well as understanding the implications of all the investigations and procedures is, to a large extent, why he is doing so well. Stephen's wisdom and insight will benefit the reader and, truth be told, would also educate health professionals as they would then get to understand what patients themselves go through during this rather arduous journey.

Medicine has "fads" like any other discipline. Stephen has taken the time to educate himself and, by means of this book, others, as to what he can do for himself to improve his well-being. It is both laudable and profoundly appreciated as his attending cardiologist. The treatment of cardiac disease has changed tremendously over the 30 years since I have graduated from medical school and will continue to change profoundly over the next 30 years, and beyond. What will not change is the need for an educated patient and for that individual to take responsibility, to a large extent, for their ongoing well-being and resultant good health and happiness. Stephen has exemplified this in spades and passes on that knowledge to the reader.

It is my honor to know and treat Stephen and now read his insightful words.

Saul Isserow, MBBCh, FRCPC, FACC
Director, VGH Centre for Cardiovascular Health
Director, Sports Cardiology BC
Director, Cardiology Services, UBC Hospital
Regional Medical Director, Vancouver Coastal Health Cardiac Rehabilitation

Dr. Gerry Ryder

I have been involved with Stephen's exploration of complementary medicine since his heart bypass surgery in January, 2009. He fortunately has ongoing excellent medical care with his family physician and cardiologist. My primary interest is to explore with patients, their own personal biological individuality – and its effect on preventative medicine and regenerative medicine.

Stephen is the perfect patient – inquisitive, intelligent, disciplined, and compliant. With this book, he is sharing with others his personal medical learning.

G. B. Ryder, B. Pharm, M.D.
Consultant in Integrative Medicine

It so happens that I share my health adventure with two of my professional colleagues and dear friends who have also contributed to the Foreword.

Dr. Bill Davis

Not many of us will escape the experience of illness or life interrupting sickness in the course of our lifetime. However, some significant numbers of us will experience a life-threatening health event at some point, and the timing and circumstances of that threat to life most assuredly will impact our chance of surviving the event.

Whether you have had a life-threatening episode or not, you can be thankful to Stephen Marks and Denise Rogers for taking the time to capture their experience. They have shared openly and honestly the significant symptom recognition and decision-making process, the physical demands, and the emotional and psychological challenges associated with surviving and recovering from a health threat that not everyone survives.

We hear people all around us, of all ages, contracting severe illness and some of them die. Many, however, are blessed and get to go on with their lives. Either outcome cannot touch us enough just by listening to prepare us for the actual magnitude of personally journeying through a life-threatening event.

I have spent the majority of my professional life having the meaningful opportunity to work with men and women during the first 24–36 hours after surviving a potentially lethal threat to life. I learned that whether the threat was to their own life or someone else's was not the key variable determining the impact of the event on their lives. Whether someone died, or could have, or even should have (given the circumstances) also does not dictate the magnitude of the journey to emotional recovery.

What is important is the significance of the person to you, or the way the threat manifested itself, or the opportunity to intervene and prevent loss of life, or the timely entry into medical care and/ or journeying together through every aspect of the ordeal. These factors so significantly impact a person's ability to successfully return to normal and the strength and quality of the relationship that is formed between the survivors.

All of my years of involvement with trauma survival and recovery have taught me that the most significant variable affecting a person's initial physical survival, and the subsequent emotional recovery after the immediate threat to life has passed is: Having had the pre-incident opportunity to place yourself cognitively and emotionally, as realistically as possible, in the potential threat before it happens.

Police officers and pilots train using simulations and simulators. It prepares them to respond physically and emotionally for what will potentially happen before it happens for real. This is both skills training and stress inoculation. Go there, be there emotionally before it happens. Other people's experiences are often the only glimpses we get for stress inoculation against the unwelcome journey of life-threatening health experiences.

Survivors of life-threatening health events have all the diagnostic traits of trauma. Their memories are vivid, triggering arousal of their Central Nervous System, with many everyday triggers that cause re-experiencing of the most difficult aspects of the experience.

Health threats have many shared elements to them: recognizing the symptoms, making the right decisions to seek assessment or being attended to emergently, undergoing medical procedures, watching and waiting helplessly during emergent medical procedures, uncertainty, medical complications, medical encounters with health professionals, waiting for a medical diagnosis or prognosis, managing the fears, attending to the demands and necessities of normal life during an overwhelming circumstance, the blessings of help experienced from unexpected sources, etc.

Allow yourself to experience the shared moments that Steve and Denise have intentionally chosen to capture for your benefit, because you can't predict when they will be a source of strength and comfort to you or someone else you may need to assist through a life-changing encounter with their own mortality.

William L. Davis, Ph.D., C. Psych.
Retired Winnipeg Police Psychologist
Open Heart Surgery Survivor

Dr. Gordon Walter

Few people have been more dedicated to a healthy and all things in moderation lifestyle than Steve. He knew and knows how to live right and does so better than 99 percent of the population. How, then, was he 'blindsided'? And let me admit that the same thing happened to me two months before this writing when a 'routine' angiogram triggered my immediate hospitalization and quadruple bypass. I can't explain it but the book might help some avoid similar rude surprises.

I can explain my current state of mind, and just how lucky I was/am to be alive today. I suddenly see myself as a "leaf in the wind" – not captain of the ship called me. The entire experience has induced a radical humility. By analogy, I used to think of myself as driving a car to my destinations. Now I realize the degree to which I have been a passenger at the back of a bus over which I have no real control. Yes, we all can choose this pair of shoes over that but when it comes to the truly massive things – like a surprising continuation of life – we are mere passengers in our journey.

This book's authors tell the simplest of stories with the most concrete, mundane daily events about one of the most profound of life's experiences. The illusion (or delusion) of 'being in control' has no cure quite like their 'tale of two perspectives'. Medical emergencies and dangers are unlike typical momentary "scares" such as while driving on an icy road. Instead, the deep truth seeps in over days and, for some, perhaps even years. The result is the realization that one is not the captain of one's own ship. Instead, one is in the back seat of the bus, a mere spectator of unfolding decisions and actions by what were only moments before complete strangers.

Perhaps the most remarkable fact to emerge from Steve and my cardiac bypass surgery stories is that they played out in the US and in Canada in such nearly identical ways. Advanced societies have advanced and highly professional medical systems populated by a virtual army of skilled and conscientious people: nurses, doctors, technology allocators, technicians, and cleaning staff. And Canada delivered the same astonishingly good care for me as the US did for Steve. Politics aside, both our 'buses' were nearly indistinguishable in design, maintenance, and performance. And we both are lucky to be living where we do.

Gordon A. Walter, Ph.D.

Introduction

This book is about saving lives, possibly yours! I was very lucky but after reading this book, you will not have to rely on luck, which we all know is very risky and undependable. You will be arming yourself with the knowledge that you need to take good care of yourself.

I was told that 20–30 percent of the population do not experience the traditional symptoms associated with heart problems. My father had his first heart attack when he was 50 years old so I grew up in a household where angina, chest pain from exertion, and nitroglycerin pills were commonplace. In addition, over the last 20 years, on every visit to my doctor, he asked me the standard questions: Do you have any chest pain, any tightness in your chest, any shortness of breath, any nausea? My answers to these questions were and continue to be NO! Even given my genetic predisposition, I would have been an unlikely candidate for heart problems if the position that its primary causes are based in lifestyle choices is true. As all my friends and associates would attest, I was a "poster boy" for living a healthy lifestyle. I exercised, watched what I ate, visited the doctor regularly and took my vitamins! However, I did have other symptoms that had unknown causes or logical explanations. This book is about my personal adventure with coronary artery disease, a condition that unfortunately, I share with millions of other citizens of the developed world.

The Format for the Book

This "adventure" is written from two perspectives. The first is from my point of view as the person who was experiencing the events directly and the second is from Denise's perspective as she accompanied me on the "journey".

Each section, where appropriate, will first describe events through my eyes and then Denise will tell you in her own words what was really happening! Her name proceeds her comments.

Our experiences were very different and highlight the importance of understanding the needs and feelings of everyone involved in the experience since they might very well not be the same.

Part 1

What are the Risks?

The risk that we are talking about here is heart disease
in all its manifestations.

Are We at Risk?

If you happen to live in a first world/developed country, then unfortunately the answer to the question "Are we at risk?" is yes. The combination of the consumption of a refined food diet, obesity, a lack of exercise and a stressful lifestyle are the "breeding conditions" for the disease. The relationship between the near epidemic proportions of cardiovascular disease and the eating habits of first world countries like the U.S., Canada, and Western Europe is undeniable. First world countries have dramatically increased the distance between the production and the consumption of food. Prior to the advent of the refined food industry, food was typically produced and consumed locally and was in its natural, unprocessed form. Today, even though food in its natural form is abundant, it competes with an enormous variety of refined foods. Unfortunately, the more you consume a diet dominated by refined foods rather than food in its natural form, the greater your risk of contracting heart disease.

Our vulnerability is further increased by one of the hallmarks of first world countries, the transition from occupations that required considerable physical activity to those that focus on mental activity. Exercising after work simply wasn't even considered after one spent a day mining, logging or working in the fields! Today, exercise for everyone that doesn't have this provided as a part of their occupation must become a planned part of the daily routine. A sedentary lifestyle is one of the contributing factors to the epidemic in heart disease.

Are You at Risk?

The answer to this question is maybe. There are a number of determining factors:

- Your Medical and Dental Health
- Medical Markers
- Weight
- Heredity or Genetic Predisposition
- Nutritional Habits
- Exercise Habits
- Personality Type
- State of Mind
- Level of Stress and
- Unhealthy "Bad Habits"

Medical and Dental Health

It's important that everyone ensure that they visit a doctor and a dentist on a regular basis. Regular should mean more frequently than every ten years or when an acute problem or emergency arises. Dental health has an important relationship to cardiovascular health in that untreated cavities and gum disease can have a negative effect on heart health.

Self-Quiz

How frequently do you pay a visit to your doctor, dentist and dental hygienist? (Author's note: I see my doctor and dentist at least once a year and my dental hygienist at least a couple times a year.)

The quiz below and those that follow are in no way intended to be considered "scientific". They are merely offered to give you an idea of your potential degree of risk.

PLACE YOURSELF ON THE SCALE BELOW

____ 0. I see my doctor and my dentist, especially my dental hygienist at least a couple times every year.

____ 1. I make sure to see my doctor and dentist at least every year.

____ 2. I visit my doctor and my dentist every two to three years unless there is a specific reason for more frequent visits.

____ 3. I had checkups within the last five years and am probably due for a follow-up with both my doctor and my dentist.

____ 4. I just see my doctor and dentist for emergencies such as a specific ailment or complaint or a broken tooth.

____ 5. I hate visits to doctors and dentists so I avoid them.

Medical Markers

There are a number of important medical markers that are used to monitor your potential risk for cardiovascular disease. All of these medical markers are related in varying degrees as well as to the sections that follow. The main ones are: Blood Pressure; Cholesterol Levels; Weight; Blood Sugar and possibly a marker for inflammation. For example, high blood pressure and/or diabetes might run in your family. These are routine tests that your family doctor would run when you have a periodic or yearly checkup and your doctor is the best source of information regarding the meaning of your numbers and the actions that are most appropriate for you to take.

I was tracking my blood pressure and cholesterol well before my January 2009 event. My cholesterol was slightly elevated, but I always chose to control it through diet rather than medication. In retrospect, this may not have been the best decision. However, there were no other indications that I was in any imminent danger. I also had a number of scans over the years, which failed to identify any problems. I believed that I was doing everything that I needed to be doing to take care of myself.

Self-Quiz

To what extent are you aware of your numbers?

PLACE YOURSELF ON THE SCALE BELOW

___ 0. I know all my numbers, and they are updated at my yearly physical exam.

___ 1. I know most of my numbers and they are updated on a semi-regular schedule.

___ 2. I have my numbers monitored every two to three years unless there is a specific reason for more frequent review.

___ 3. I had a checkup a while ago and am probably due for a follow up.

___ 4. I've been told that it would be a good idea to have a physical with the accompanying blood tests but I haven't got around to it yet.

___ 5. I feel fine so what's the point?

Since weight is such a crucial "number" with so many implications it is measured separately.

Self-Quiz

To what extent do you track your weight?

PLACE YOURSELF ON THE SCALE BELOW

___ 0. I weigh myself daily and keep it within a healthy range.

___ 1. My weight is stable and within a healthy range.

___ 2. My weight is relatively stable and when it gets above a certain point I take steps to lose a few pounds.

___ 3. I'm slightly overweight and am taking steps to lose some pounds.

___ 4. I'm moderately overweight and periodically attempt to take steps to lose some pounds.

___ 5. I know I'm significantly overweight but I don't pay any attention to it.

Heredity or Genetic Predisposition

Is there heart disease in your family? If so, who? The answer to this question is a great clue to whether this factor relates to you.

My father's older brother died in his fifties from heart related issues and my father had his first heart attack when he was 50 years old. He survived that event and another one a year later and lived another 24 years. I reduced the importance of this information because there were dramatic differences between my lifestyle and that of my father's. I believed that a healthy lifestyle could more than compensate for a genetic predisposition. As will be discussed, this turned out to be only partially true.

Self-Quiz

To what extent is your hereditary/genetic blueprint an issue?

PLACE YOURSELF ON THE SCALE BELOW

___ 0. To my knowledge there is no one on my father or mother's sides of the family with any history of heart disease.

___ 1. Either my father or mother have one or two ancestors with a history of heart disease.

___ 2. Both my father and mother have one or two ancestors with a history of heart disease.

___ 3. There is significant evidence of heart disease on one or both sides of my parents' families.

___ 4. One of my parents and one of my siblings have heart disease.

___ 5. Both my parents and one or more of my siblings have heart disease.

Nutritional Habits

Whether or not you are at risk from a nutritional perspective depends to a large part on the extent to which you participate in the "fast food lifestyle". Are you into burgers, French fries, pizza, commercially baked goods, and so on? You get the idea. The more you consume a diet dominated by refined foods rather than food in its natural form, the greater your risk of contracting heart disease.

Growing up I ate my share of burgers, pizza and French fries but as I grew older I gradually gravitated to a diet that increased the proportion of food in its natural form and reduced the amount of "fast" or "junk" food. One of the comments that my cardiologist made post-event was that my healthy lifestyle probably prolonged the onset of my problem and reduced its severity.

Self-Quiz

To what extent is your eating behavior an issue?

PLACE YOURSELF ON THE SCALE BELOW

___ 0. I never eat junk food and rarely consume refined foods. My diet consists almost exclusively of food in its natural, unprocessed form.

___ 1. I rarely eat junk food and occasionally consume refined foods. My diet consists mostly of food in its natural, unprocessed form.

___ 2. I occasionally eat junk food and sometimes consume refined foods. My diet consists mostly of food in its natural, unprocessed form.

____ 3. I sometimes eat junk food and sometimes consume refined foods. My diet consists often of food in its natural, unprocessed form.

____ 4. I frequently eat junk food and consume refined foods. My diet on occasion consists of food in its natural, unprocessed form, but this is something that I do not pay much attention to.

____ 5. I frequently eat junk food and consume refined foods. I do not pay much attention to what or how much I eat.

Exercise Habits

Whether or not you are at risk from an exercise perspective depends on how active you are. To what extent do you fall victim to a sedentary lifestyle? Are you a "couch potato", a "fitness fanatic", or a "weekend warrior"? For the most part, when we were young, we were constantly moving. However, as we transition from childhood, adolescence and young adulthood to an adult lifestyle our level of physical activity diminishes. Whereas physical activity was an integral part of "growing up", as adults we have to make a focused effort to incorporate physical activity into our daily routine. This is a challenge that many people fail to meet. The basic principle here is somewhat parallel to the one discussed above for nutrition: The more physically active you are, the healthier you will be. Our bodies were meant to move! The type of exercise or activity is much less important than the degree to which you live at the active end of the sedentary/active continuum, which is represented in the quiz below.

After being fairly active athletically as I was growing up, I went through a 15 to 20 year period when I did not have any systematic exercise regime. In my mid-forties I discovered power walking, which has led me to become a devotee of the 10,000 steps a day approach to fitness. In addition, I adopted the practice of doing pushups since maintaining muscle mass and strength is increasingly important as we get older.

Self-Quiz

To what extent is your exercise behavior an issue?

PLACE YOURSELF ON THE SCALE BELOW

___ 0. A variety of aerobic and strengthening exercise is a regular part of my routine. I exercise at least 3–5 times a week or more.

___ 1. I know that exercise is important and I consistently participate in some physical activity at least 3 times a week.

___ 2. I know that exercise is important but my schedule and other commitments prevent me from consistently participating in some physical activity. However, I usually find time to exercise at least 1 or 2 times a week.

___ 3. I know that exercise is important but my schedule and other commitments prevent me from consistently participating in some physical activity. However, I usually find time to exercise at least 4 times a month.

___ 4. I do not consciously think about exercise and assume that the activity involved in my regular daily routine is sufficient.

___ 5. I do not do any form of "formal" exercise as well as choosing to ride rather than walk as an option of getting from point A to point B. Relaxation for me is lying on the couch and watching my favorite TV shows.

Personality Type

One's personality is also a potential risk factor in terms of cardio-vascular disease. There are many different ways of approaching this discussion. In the service of simplicity, a description of the "Type A" personality contrasted with the "Type B" personality will illustrate this point. Type A's are demanding, hard driving, impatient, and quick to anger. They tend to be "highly strung". These individuals are at greater risk of contracting heart disease. On the other hand, Type B's lack the sense of urgency displayed by type A's and they tend to be more easygoing, understanding, and patient than their aggressive counterparts. If you are in doubt about which type best describes you, ask a few close family members or colleagues at work, and they will tell you! Armed with this information answer the quiz below.

My personal profile runs counter to the theme above. I fall clearly into the Type B category. I tend not to possess or display the characteristics of a Type A personality beyond what would be normal expressions of emotion and behavior in the course of day-to-day activities.

Self-Quiz

Which personality type best describes you? For the purpose of this quiz we will look at relative percentages rather than being absolutely one type or the other.

PLACE YOURSELF ON THE SCALE BELOW
___ 0. I am a 90%+ Type B.
___ 1. I am 65–89% Type B.
___ 2. I am 50–64% Type B.
___ 3. I am 50–64% Type A.

___ 4. I am 65–89% Type A.
___ 5. I am 90%+ Type A.

State of Mind

There are several different ways of approaching this category. They are: Worldview; Mental Practices; and Lifestyle Stress.

Worldview

Are you an optimist or a pessimist? This refers to whether your expectations for how things will turn out are positive or negative. Do you walk with a smile or have a raincloud over your head? Do you look at what can go right or what can go wrong? Do you believe that things have a way of working out or do you worry constantly about potential negative outcomes? Do you know someone who is an optimist? What is it like to have them around? Conversely, do you know someone who is a pessimist? What is it like to be in their company?

I do my share of worrying and anticipating events that never happen, but when push comes to shove usually expect a positive outcome. I wouldn't classify myself as a "model optimist", but I am certainly not a "model pessimist".

Self-Quiz

To what degree are you an optimist or a pessimist? As above, for the purpose of this quiz we will also look at relative percentages rather than being absolutely one or the other.

PLACE YOURSELF ON THE SCALE BELOW

___ 0. I am a 90%+ Optimist.

___ 1. I am 65–89% Optimist.

___ 2. I am 50–64% Optimist.

___ 3. I am 50–64% Pessimist.

___ 4. I am 65–89% Pessimist.

___ 5. I am 90%+ Pessimist.

Mental Practices

There are a number of mental practices that one can engage in to mitigate the contributing factors of cardiovascular disease. These include meditation, spending quiet and/or contemplative time, relaxing, or becoming engaged in any activity that takes you "away" from your daily stresses. Do you routinely participate in one or more of these activities? Is starting or ending the day sitting quietly a part of your routine, or something that you've never done? When was the last time you took a walk in the park? Do you find getting lost in a good book rejuvenating?

Here's where walking serves a dual purpose. I find that being out in nature on a regular basis with no agenda other than getting some exercise is something that is relaxing and clears my mind.

Self-Quiz

To what degree are one or more of the above mental practices a part of your life?

PLACE YOURSELF ON THE SCALE BELOW

___ 0. These practices are an indispensable part of my daily routine.

___ 1. Several of these practices are a regular part of my weekly routine.

___ 2. A few of these practices are a hit or miss part of my weekly routine.

___ 3. A few of these practices might be a part of my monthly routine.

___ 4. A walk in the park or recreational reading is an infrequent activity.

___ 5. These practices and I are strangers; our paths rarely cross.

Add your score for Worldview and Mental Practices and divide by two. This will be your score for State of Mind.

Worldview ____ + Mental Practices ____ /2 = ____ TOTAL "STATE OF MIND" SCORE

Lifestyle Stress

The degree of stress in our lives is another potential contributing risk factor. This stress comes from many sources: Relationships; Finances; Work (including the commute); and the unpredictable emergencies that randomly appear such as a physical injury or an automobile accident. Is your family life happy and tranquil or volatile and tumultuous? For most of us reality is some combination of the two extremes. The question is the proportion of the "calm" and the "stressful". Are financial concerns constantly on your mind? Are you worried about how the bills are going to be paid? Or does stress here come from a business venture or investment that appears to be in jeopardy? At work, are you worried about the demands of a particular task or assignment that you are finding challenging? Or maybe there are conflicts with coworkers or your boss?

Is the culture of your workplace positive or toxic? What is the frequency of the "unexpected" in your life? Do you find your normal routine is frequently interrupted by emergencies that are distressing and distracting?

I attempt to reduce the amount of stress in my life, but I am regularly visited by work deadlines resulting from my own procrastination, periodic normally occurring relationship misunderstandings along with the anxiety accompanying unsuccessful attempts to predict the stock market.

Self-Quiz

To what extent is the stress in your life an issue? No attempt is made to distinguish among the different sources for stress as briefly outlined above. This task is left to you, the reader, to assess the average amount of stress that you deal with and respond accordingly.

PLACE YOURSELF ON THE SCALE BELOW

___ 0. My life is relatively free of stress aside from what one would normally encounter as a part of one's daily routine.

___ 1. Usually, my life is relatively free of stress aside from what one would normally encounter as a part of one's daily routine.

___ 2. Occasionally, my life is relatively free of stress aside from what one would normally encounter as a part of one's daily routine.

___ 3. I cope regularly with at least one of the above stressors in my life.

___ 4. I cope regularly with more than one of the above stressors in my life.

___ 5. I cope regularly with several or more of the above stressors in my life.

Unhealthy "Bad" Habits

There are a number of additional factors that raise the probability of contracting cardiovascular disease. These are smoking, alcohol consumption, fast food and living a stressful lifestyle. These last two have already been addressed in the Nutritional Habits, Exercise Habits and Lifestyle Stress sections, but are repeated here for emphasis. The abuse of prescription, non-prescription and illegal drugs is a bad habit that will not be addressed. If the latter happens to be an issue for you, reading this book is like moving deck chairs on the Titanic!

The first one is smoking. Regardless of how compelling advertising campaigns of the past for smoking may have been, smoking is a "nasty" habit, which will compromise your health! If you smoke, stop immediately! If you don't smoke, absolutely don't consider starting!

The second bad habit is drinking alcohol. Even though alcohol consumption is inextricably woven into our social fabric, moderation is definitely the standard to follow. The problem here is that people who have the problem don't see it. Are you a "social" drinker? Remember that there is a fine line between being a "social" drinker and being a "functioning" alcoholic! If you drink, do so moderately, which is defined as a few times a week. If you drink occasionally, that's not a problem. If you don't drink, don't consider starting!

The more that fast foods form a regular part of your diet, the greater the problem. And yes, unfortunately, pizza is fast food, even if it has veggies on it. Lifestyle stress is created by the absence of exercise and positive mindfulness activities accompanied by poor time management, stressful relationships, and financial problems. Every effort should be made to minimize and/or remove these negative stressors from your life.

An example of "Do what I say not what I do" is illustrated, at times, by my snacking behavior after dinner during which I will consume my three small squares of chocolate along with a few cookies. Eating the whole box of cookies was never a problem, and I am able to limit my cookie count, but would probably be better off without them at all.

Self-Quiz

In responding to this scale, simply take an average over the four bad habits to establish which category best describes you:

PLACE YOURSELF ON THE SCALE BELOW
___ 0. I don't have any bad habits.
___ 1. I very rarely might be guilty of one or two of the bad habits.
___ 2. I periodically might be guilty of one or two of the bad habits.
___ 3. I frequently might be guilty of one or more of the bad habits.
___ 4. I frequently might be guilty of more than one of the bad habits.
___ 5. When I look at the list of bad habits, I see myself everywhere!

Scoring the Quiz

Record your score for each of the categories below in the space provided.

Medical and Dental Health ____
Medical Markers ____
Weight ____
Heredity or Genetic Predisposition ____
Nutritional Habits ____
Exercise Habits ____
Personality Type ____
State of Mind ____
Lifestyle Stress____
Unhealthy "Bad" Habits____
Total____

Key

- 0–15 points: Congratulations! You're in good shape. Keep it up!
- 16–25 points: You are in fairly good shape. Focus on the categories where you can improve most and start a program to do so.
- 26–35 points: You have considerable room for improvement. Focus on the categories where you can improve most and start a program to do so.
- 36+ points: The horns are sounding and the sirens are ringing, and no, this is not a celebration! Your scores on the quiz indicate that you have much work to do to reduce your risks. Start with the categories that you scored the highest on and begin. It's more important to take action and less important where you start.

There is considerable information included at the end of the book to help you in your quest to reduce your risks.

Part 2

A Time Line of the Events

BEFORE DEPARTURE

The Donated TV

I simply hate to see waste. In the fall of 2008, I attended one of my client's golf tournaments and to my delight and surprise, I won the "grand prize", which was a home entertainment system including a 40" Sony TV. Consequently, the 19-year-old 27-incher was now obsolete. We found a good home for it and two of the staff at the Neighborhood House were coming by to take it away on the morning of December 5th. It was really heavy, and I volunteered to help carry it down the stairs and put it in their SUV.

Denise: I was out at the time and didn't see the "spectacle". I thought Steve would not be carrying the TV down the stairs. It was so heavy. When I got home and he told me what he had done, I was quite concerned.

A Trip to the Doctor

I didn't have any problems carrying the TV down the stairs. However, afterwards I just didn't feel very well. No pain or shortness of breath, just a feeling of not being quite right. So, it was off to my doctor to get checked out. He gave me a cardiogram (EKG) and took some blood tests to check for the signs of heart damage. My EKG was normal for me, and the blood tests were negative so he gave me the "good to go" for our flight to Maui, which left the following Monday.

Denise: With our trip to Maui pending, I hoped Steve would be OK. Deep down, I was also sorry we had to miss, for the second year in a row, the annual Christmas luncheon with Steve's group of TEC Chairs and their spouses. But, but, but we make it a point to see our doctors if anything feels weird and "not quite right". I was thankful Steve received the "go ahead" from his doctor. Strange though, I had this underlying feeling, maybe intuition, that something was going to happen.

HOLIDAY TIME

Our Regular Routine

We have taken a winter break in Maui most years since 1989. We go to the same unit in a delightful older complex right on the water in the Napili area north of Lahaina. We walk, shop, cook, read, and generally just hang out in that warm, gentle environment. The break renews and invigorates us.

A typical day would be as follows: Up fairly early. Breakfast – A protein shake for me and oat bran porridge for Denise unless it was

Sunday, which would mean "healthy pancakes"! Then we would drive up to the Kapalua Resort, park by the church, and walk for about an hour along the fairways of the Bay Course and through the Norfolk Pines. Spectacular!

We would then come back to the unit, have a bite to eat and a rest before going into Lahaina to shop for dinner. In the afternoon, we might walk again ostensibly to look for golf balls and then return to our unit to prepare dinner. Cooking is one of my hobbies, and we discovered a long time ago that the best food is always prepared by our own hands.

In the evening, we would read, watch some TV, rent a movie or once in a while, go into town to the theatre. This is a routine that we have never tired of. And aside from being a bit "tired", this year was no different than any of the past ones. There were no clues of what was to come!

I just kept having this feeling of "what is going to happen next", given that shortly into the trip I had to visit the doctor for a routine matter.

The Big Island

One of the "departures" from our usual routine was our attendance at the Creativity and Madness Conference, a sanctioned professional development event for people in the health professions, mainly psychiatrists, physicians, psychologists, and social workers. The Conference explores the relationship between the Arts and Helping Professions. This year, the conference was being held on the Big Island at the Hilton Waikoloa Resort. I was presenting at the conference. An added bonus to the trip was the opportunity to connect with one of my past graduate students who is a psychologist on the Island. The hassle of extricating ourselves from "paradise" was balanced by the opportunity to explore some new places, for some intellectual stimulation, and the chance to reconnect with a dear friend.

I was not particularly interested in packing up again to attend the conference but there was really no choice. The fact that I was not feeling well did not help. I would have preferred to stay on Maui!

Presenting at the Conference

I am a Counselling Psychologist by training, specializing in Group Process and Experiential Learning. My presentation at the Conference was focused on providing an opportunity for the attendees to meet each other and make connections with those people with whom they had common interests. It was a bit like "herding cats" but feedback nevertheless was very positive. The participants made connections that simply would not have happened without the event.

Looking back on this experience, which was not without its stressful moments, is very interesting given the events that were on the immediate horizon!

Denise: I just remember Steve being so tired. We just wanted to get back to our condo on Maui!

Returning to the "Cove"

The conference ended on December 31, and we wanted to return to Maui as soon as we could. The flight back took us through Honolulu, which turned a 20-minute flight into a four hour "adventure".

Once again, there were heavy suitcases to maneuver along with the general stress associated with traveling. I was glad to get back to the Cove – to get back home!

THE "ADVENTURE" BEGINS

Some Very Bad Eating Choices

The complex where we stay has a tradition of hosting a New Year's Eve dinner for all the guests. When we arrived, the food had been picked over but there were still an abundance of deep fried chicken wings and cold chow mein. We were both very hungry, and I also have great difficulty passing on "free food"! This confluence of events resulted in me consuming two large helpings of the wings and noodles! I realized that it was a mistake while I was eating but my hunger ruled. This behavior was completely out of character for me since I never eat deep fried chicken wings! Needless to say, I did not feel very well after dinner.

One of our New Year's traditions is to go out for dinner on January 1st. This year we were planning to go to Ruth's Chris Steak House, but we decided to postpone our celebration to the next day. A meal at Ruth's was way more than I could handle based on my prior evening's indiscretions. Instead, we opted for pot roast sandwiches at home but again, I found a way to add to my already upset stomach. My eyes were bigger than my stomach, and I forced down two sand-wiches, which in retrospect was one too many!

The next evening it was off to Ruth's. The steak arrived floating in melted butter so it was sent back to the kitchen. However, the mashed potatoes were also heavily buttered, but we did not have the will to return it as well. It was a great dinner but much richer food than we were accustomed to.

Denise: Ditto!

"Indigestion"

Over the next few days, I had a mild case of indigestion, which was very easily explained in my mind. I was just not feeling very well. However, the thing that was different this time is it did not go away. On Wednesday, January 7th, I was still not feeling right so Denise insisted that I should go to the West Maui Medical Clinic the following morning if I was not feeling better. I reluctantly agreed, but I really did not see the need.

Denise: I thought it best for Steve to see the doctor and allay my fears and any he might have as to how he was feeling.

Thursday Morning and it's off to the Clinic

I had mixed feelings about going to the clinic. On the one hand, I realized that it was the prudent thing to do even though I knew that there was nothing fundamentally wrong. But on the other hand, I was a bit frightened that the trip might lead to more tests and hassle, which I preferred to avoid. I never considered that there might be a serious problem.

At the clinic, I was given an EKG and my blood was tested for the enzymes that were markers for heart damage. My blood test came back negative but Dr. Azman did not like the looks of my cardiogram and decided not to take any chances. He ordered up an ambulance to take me to Emergency at Maui Memorial on the east side of the Island. It's about a 45-minute ride. I told him that I felt fine and was up to driving myself but he questioned why I would want to do that and insisted on the ambulance. Denise would follow in our rental car. So much for avoiding the hassle! However, I still believed nothing was wrong.

Dr. Azman became the second person who saved my life. Denise was the first by insisting that I go to the clinic, an action I would not have initiated on my own. It would have been very easy for him to send me home attributing my problem to indigestion, which would dissipate.

Denise: I was really concerned for Steve because of what he said to me when Dr. Azman was out of the room. He was in tears and stated that his greatest fear was having a heart event, which appeared to be coming true. The doctor did an EKG on Steve and didn't like the results so he gave him an Aspirin and sent him to the hospital in an ambulance.

I felt frightened, frantic, like my whole world was starting to fall apart. As I walked to the car to follow, although the ambulance was already well on its way, a woman approached me and asked if I needed help. She was one of the many angels that would appear to help me. I felt kind of numb and mumbled, "I was all right," and got into the car to drive to the other side of the Island, which I had never done on my own.

An Ambulance Ride to Emergency

We had driven the road many times but I never saw it from this perspective, looking out the back window! The paramedics were excellent and did all they could to make me comfortable. If a ride in an ambulance could ever be considered "pleasant", this one would qualify. At this point, I was more frustrated with our day being interfered with than I was concerned about myself. We arrived at the hospital without event, and I was admitted.

Denise: My ride was anything but pleasant, but thankfully also uneventful. I just moved with the traffic and was able to find Maui Memorial Hospital quite easily from the directions that the ambulance drivers provided. I parked the car and went to find Steve.

The Day in Emergency

The experience in Emergency was not unlike what one would expect anywhere. The facility was busy but not overwhelmed. Nevertheless, it took a few hours for one of the attending physicians to visit. I was X-rayed, given another EKG, and a series of blood tests. Efforts were made to have my most recent cardiograms sent from Vancouver. Then there was a fair amount of waiting. My X-rays and blood tests came back normal and the cardiogram was not that different than the ones sent from home.

Denise: Contrary to the tone of Steve's description above, I found this time extremely stressful. It brought me back to being in Emergency on separate occasions with both my mother and father when they were at the end of their lives. And also, even though we knew Maui well, we had no support system. I felt truly alone.

An Echocardiogram and a Stress Test

As a final procedure, it was decided to give me an echocardiogram and a stress test before making the final decision to discharge me. The echocardiogram was administered without event, but the attending cardiologist, Dr. Pamela Gordon, saw some things that concerned her, and she decided not to put me on the treadmill. Now, for the first time, I was becoming concerned.

I then met with Dr. Ben Massenburg, the Emergency Physician, and he said that they were going to fly me on an air ambulance into Honolulu and refer me to the Straub Medical Center for further observation. He chose this facility since it specialized in cardiac-related issues. Any illusion that our lives were quickly going to revert to normal had now disappeared.

Dr. Ben Massenburg and Dr. Pamela Gordon became the third and fourth people whose actions saved my life. Had they not taken the conservative approach and instead sent me home, my life would have unfolded, or should I say, unraveled, much differently. However, this was unknown to me at the time.

Denise: All I can remember at the time was taking Dr. Gordon aside and asking her if Steve was going to be all right. Her response was, "Yes, he'll be fine. Just don't let him see you upset." Dr. Massenburg also took me aside and suggested that I go back to our condo and pack everything up and then go to Honolulu. However, I was not interested in leaving Steve at this point. We did not know what was going to happen. I wanted to fly in the air ambulance with him to Honolulu. We were not sure if packing up the condo was even necessary. It certainly was not a priority at this point.

An Ambulance Ride to the Airport

Any illusion that January the 8th was going to revert to a normal holiday day was now completely gone! The thought did run through my mind that I had the option of declining the trip to Honolulu and returning to the Cove, but who am I to argue with three doctors? I put my faith in them and chose to believe that they knew what they were doing.

We left our rental car at the hospital with assurances that it would be safe there, and Denise and I took the short ambulance ride to the airport. It was comforting having her with me. It was now dark, and I was probably in a mild state of shock. Consequently, I have no clear memories of this part of my journey. It was simply another uneventful ambulance ride.

Denise: I also have no clear recollection of that ride either. At this point, I'm sure that I was also in shock. This part of the experience is just a blur.

An Air Ambulance Ride to Honolulu

The transfer to the air ambulance was seamless. As I recall, there were two nurses and the pilot. It was a very small plane and there was barely room for all of us. As an indicator of how much I was "out of it" at this point, the nurses were successful in selling us a one-year insurance policy to cover the cost of the flight and any further flights in the event that there was a shortfall between our travel insurance and the cost of the service – $99.00. When we returned to Vancouver, I was able to get the $99.00 refunded from the company since if I was in my right mind I would never have purchased the policy in the first place!

The flight into Honolulu was uneventful as well. Aside from a growing sense of apprehension, I felt fine; I was not in any discomfort.

Denise: It wasn't certain if I could even fly over in the Air Ambulance with Steve. At the hospital the nurse asked, "What's your weight?" "One hundred thirty pounds." I said. "I think we can fit you in," which is what they did. I was so grateful that I could fly with Steve and not have to wait until the next morning for a commercial flight.

That would have meant an hour's drive on a dark mountain highway back to the condo and spending the night alone not knowing what was happening.

It was a very small plane ... the pilot, two nurses, Steve on a gurney and me flying across the dark Pacific. God, I prayed that we'd make it to Honolulu! My anxiety level was off the chart!

An Ambulance Ride to the Straub Medical Center

If I was unable to recall much detail related to the ambulance ride from Maui Memorial to the airport in Kahului, I can remember even less of this one! It was a relatively quick ride that proceeded without event.

Denise: A half-hour flight and we arrived. The tarmac was empty. I felt disoriented. Another ambulance was waiting. The attendants loaded Steve in the back, and I sat up front. We were driven to the Straub Center in downtown Honolulu. Steve was taken directly to a room. I could stay overnight with him the nurse reassured us. The cardiologist was on his way. Dr. Kai arrived within the hour and told us he would do an angiogram in the morning. I was numb!

Getting "Tucked in" on 3 West – The Cardiac Care Ward

Upon arriving at the hospital, I was taken directly to the Cardiac Care Ward, 3 West. I can't remember the exact time but I am guessing it was around 9:00 p.m. There was already paperwork there for me so Maui Memorial and Straub had been in communication. I was taken to a private room and put into bed. I recall a sense of relief as

I relaxed in bed. I had survived the ordeal of being transported to Honolulu unscathed and was now in the best place I could be. Aside from the underlying apprehension and being a bit tired from the trip, I still felt fine.

The nursing staff were all friendly, accommodating, and demonstrated a real and genuine interest in me. I was kept fairly busy with the set-up for being monitored. I was prepared for IV drips and blood was taken along with an EKG. This was the beginning of what would be a regular routine. Denise wanted to stay with me so they made the large reclining chair in the room up into a bed. All that remained now was to wait for the cardiologist.

Dr. Massenburg had told me that he chose to refer me to Straub since they specialized in cardiac issues. Upon arriving at the hospital, I discovered that Straub was the hospital that was the referral destination for all complex cardiac cases in the Pacific Rim. I truly was in the right place, even though I did not know why.

Denise: I too was relieved to see that Steve was in good hands and that I could stay with him overnight. The nurse even gave me pajamas and a toothbrush. She was so reassuring when she said, "Dr. Kai, the cardiologist is great."

A Visit from My Cardiologist – Dr. Kai

Denise and I passed the time talking about how dramatically our lives had changed in the last ten hours and reassured each other that I was in good hands. During this conversation, Dr. Kai appeared. He had a soft, calming style, which immediately put me at ease. The nurses all said that he was terrific. He made sure that I was comfortable, checked my vital signs, and told me that he would see me in the morning and that they would perform an angiogram. This procedure would provide some definitive answers as to what, if anything, was actually going on with me.

As a final note, I did not look sick in any way. Denise kept commenting that she could not believe how good I looked! The nurses were kind enough to round up something for us to eat, and we settled in for the night.

Denise: After Dr. Kai left, the nurse turned to Steve and said, "He'll probably use stents for your blocked arteries. You'll be fine and able to travel back to Maui to finish your holiday." I felt so grateful that our lives would soon return to "normal".

Friday Morning and it's off for an Angiogram

The night was uneventful. Apart from being awakened for blood tests, blood pressure readings or EKGs at intervals throughout the night, I actually slept! The morning started at around 5:30 a.m. After a few hours, a nurse's aide from the OR came to transport me. I can remember being transferred into the OR, having Dr. Kai explain the procedure to me, and then being heavily sedated but conscious. The procedure was painless and was over quite quickly. I was then returned to the ward.

When I was admitted to the hospital, I thought that it would be a good idea to keep a daily journal of the events but unfortunately I simply did not have whatever it would have taken to do this. So much for honorable intentions!

Denise: When Steve went for the angiogram, I quickly dressed in my shorts and T-shirt I had worn the day before. We had no change of clothes or toiletries with us. I then went to the cafeteria for breakfast.

I was still feeling reassured that it would be a "simple fix" although deep down I felt anxious.

The "Bad News"!

As I had mentioned, I did not look sick. Dr. Kai was optimistic that I would be fine. Neither he nor I were expecting what came next. The results of the angiogram revealed that I had several major blockages in my main arteries, 95 percent, 90 percent, and 70 percent. It is a wonder that I never experienced any of the traditional symptoms of heart problems. It is also a wonder that I did not have an "event" given the level of my activities – push-ups, 10,000 steps a day, exercising with hand weights and carrying heavy suitcases, not to mention taking the TV down the stairs before we left!

I was well beyond angioplasty or stents. I was informed that it was a quadruple bypass for me. I was numb. My second worst fear had been realized, the first being having a heart attack and being in pain. Denise and I grieved, consoled each other, and reassured ourselves that we were in good hands.

Now that my true condition was known, I was put on a nitro drip and monitored very closely. A side effect of this medication was headaches so I was introduced to my "friend" Percocet (oxycodone HCL) with whom I would form a fast friendship for the next two months!

Denise: I was just finishing my cereal and banana when Steve was wheeled back into the room. Surprised to see him back so soon from the procedure, I asked him, "How did it go?" He mouthed the words "quadruple bypass". "What?" I said. I could not believe it. My mind reeled thinking of everything at once: Steve's operation, getting back to Maui, packing up all our belongings in the condo, returning the rental car. It felt so huge. Dr. Kai came in the room to show us the pictures from the angiogram of his blocked arteries.

His father had his first heart attack at fifty so that was a risk factor along with Steve's borderline cholesterol levels. I was so overwhelmed hearing the diagnosis and knowing what I had to do.

I asked him if it was best for me to leave and go back to Maui that afternoon. He agreed and gave me the phone number for Hawaiian Airlines.

I couldn't have felt more alone. How was I going to do it? Then I was asked to meet with one of the clerks in the billing department. One of her questions was, "Do you know your husband's wishes regarding life support?" I mumbled, "I have no idea." I returned to Steve's room and made arrangements to return to Maui.

I had just enough cash for the cab ride to the airport, couldn't get the ATM at the hospital to work so hoped that when I landed on Maui, I could use my MasterCard for the ride from the airport to Maui Memorial where I would retrieve our rental car.

Taking Care of Life's Necessary Details

Now that we knew the lay of the land, there was no longer any prospect of us returning to Maui. Consequently, the responsibility of "closing up shop" fell to Denise. She was really torn; she knew that she had to go but did not want to leave me.

She was faced with flying back to Kahului, picking up our car at Maui Memorial, driving back to our unit in Napili, packing up and settling up, returning the rental car and then flying back to Honolulu. All this was on top of dealing with all her feelings and concerns about me. We said goodbye. I told her she would be just fine and would see her Saturday afternoon.

Denise: It was so hard for me to leave. I had to "dig deep" and draw on my inner strength to keep me going. There was nothing else I could do, I had no other options, I had to keep going. I think my inner strength and resourcefulness developed when I learned how to be alone and survive when I lived in Toronto for three years.

When it was time to leave for the airport, I kissed Stephen goodbye while fighting back the tears. His nurse accompanied me downstairs and to a waiting taxi. As Steve mentioned before, the level of care was outstanding at Straub. Again, my head was just whirling; I was so stressed and anxious, not just about leaving Steve, but now worrying about catching my plane.

It was midday, so the traffic was not too bad. I arrived at the airport in plenty of time and rushed over to line up for check-in. Unfortunately, I did not have my passport with me, only my driver's license and birth certificate. My carry-on consisted of my purse and a hospital plastic bag with a few items including the DVD we rented on Maui and had not yet had a chance to return. The ticket agent stamped my boarding pass with what I found out later was a code, which singled me out for an additional security check. When I got to security, I was told to stand to the right and wait. The security officer questioned the validity of my driver's license because he had never seen one like it before. I explained that it was a license issued by the Province of British Columbia in Canada. This additional hassle really added to my anxiety. I asked him if I was going to make my plane. He said, "You might."

As it turned out, the security search went quite smoothly, and I walked quickly to the gate where I found a pay phone and called Steve to tell him that I made it safely to the airport. The flight left on time.

Meeting the Surgeon

Later that morning, I was visited by Dr. Mark Grattan, the surgeon who was going to perform the operation. He was calm, friendly, matter of fact and definitely inspired confidence. Most importantly, I learned that he was a "real pro", having performed thousands of procedures. Now I ask you, if you had to have an operation, whom would you prefer to have performing it – the doctor who was just learning, one who had completed hundreds or one who had completed thousands!

Dr. Grattan talked me through the operation and informed me that it was a procedure not without significant risks. He told me that, based on his track record, there was a two percent chance that I would not survive the operation. However, he was quick to add that apart from my coronary artery disease, I was healthy and would be just fine. I was tentatively scheduled for surgery that afternoon.

Denise: I did not have the opportunity to meet Dr. Grattan because I was en route to Maui.

"ET" Phone Home!

The only activity that I seemed to have any interest in plus the energy for was using the phone. I had a line in my room and was permitted to use it whenever I wanted. Here is a partial list of the people I called after my arrival at the hospital: my brother Les in Mexico, my cousin Gary in Vancouver, Monte Glanzberg, my doctor in Vancouver, my TEC colleague Joff, a few of the staff in the TEC office in Calgary, and our friends Nancy, Mickey, and Emily in Hawaii.

Talking to people became my way of coming to terms with my circumstances as well as a means of insulating myself from the grim realities of what I was facing. The phone became my escape, which apart from conducting the odd bit of necessary business, might explain why I had so much energy for the activity.

A Visit from Nancy and Mickey

While Denise was travelling to Maui, Nancy and Mickey stopped by to see me. It was great to have visitors! I taught with Nancy for many years at The University of British Columbia and after she retired and moved with her husband to Honolulu, we have kept in close touch. She and Denise have also become good friends. We have a tradition of reuniting with them every year when we come to Hawaii. It was wonderful to have dear friends close at hand, especially when you really need them! (Unfortunately, Dr. Mickey Slakter died in June of 2018.)

Denise: The trip to Maui passed quickly. I spoke to the man sitting beside me who I discovered was visiting Maui for a medical conference. He was a doctor, and he reassured me that quadruple bypass surgery is routine so not to worry. I was so thankful to hear that from an independent source. He was another one of the many "angels" who crossed my path during this time.

I landed at the Kahului airport. As I was short on cash, I phoned our rental car agency, which was five minutes from the airport, and asked if someone could pick me up and take me to Maui Memorial where our rental car was parked. The rep said, "We don't do that." So I walked over to the taxi stand, requested a cab that would accept MasterCard and was driven to the hospital. There was the car sitting in the lot across from the Emergency entrance. I reflected on how much our lives had changed overnight!

Now I had to make the one hour drive to the west side of the Island. Steve and I had driven this road together so many times. Here I was again driving it by myself. Ordinarily, I loved watching the ocean on these drives but today, I did not even notice it. I just kept moving towards my target – getting back to the condo.

Finally, I was turning left off the highway at the Napili exit but before I could "go home", I stopped at the shopping mall to mail a letter and return the DVD. Completing these small errands gave me a sense of normalcy in my world, which was anything but normal!

The Health Travel Insurance "Drama"

The hospital was in touch with the health travel insurance company since any procedures would have to have their prior approval before they could be performed, especially a high ticket item like a bypass. There were a series of phone calls and messages but no approvals. My surgery was postponed.

Denise: When I got back to our condo in Maui, I felt safe again. I was finally home. We've spent so much time there over the past twenty years that it is like a second home. And people rallied around me to help. I pulled into the parking lot at Honokeana Cove and Su, the rental manager, immediately came out and hugged me. We had called her earlier that day from Honolulu to tell her what happened. She asked me, "How can I help?" I replied, "I don't know where to start. I have to pack and return to Honolulu tomorrow, Saturday." I went to our condo, called Steve to tell him that I had arrived safely, then heard a knock at the door.

Mel, the Resident Manager's wife, stood at the door asking if I needed help packing. I accepted her offer, and we began. Again, another angel had appeared! "Would you stay overnight with me?"

I asked. Without hesitation, she nodded and said, "I just need to get dinner ready for Dave and my daughter, and I'll bring my sleeping bag for the couch." She left and then there was another knock at the door. This time, it was Paula Green from #203 – our next door neighbor. Su had phoned her and told her the story. Paula offered, "My husband Jim and I can help you tomorrow to return the rental car and drive you to the airport." I hesitated at first then decided the last thing that I needed was worrying about breaking down on the highway. I was so grateful for their help. Two more angels had appeared!

I slept fitfully and awoke at five thirty in the morning. Mel was up and off to work. I stood in the living room looking out at Honokeana Cove, the water was still, and this deep feeling of 'everything will be okay' came over me. I just knew Steve would be fine.

Waiting for "Authorization"

The balance of the weekend was spent in limbo waiting for the hospital to receive authorization. The issue was financial. The insurance company's position was that I would be flown back to Vancouver and have the operation performed there. They were actively looking for a bed for me. This is where Dr. Kai intervened. The nurses told me about a "conversation" he had with the insurance company in which he told them I was unstable and under no circumstances could I be moved.

Personally, I was terrified of the prospect of a six-hour flight in a small jet back to Vancouver. Absolutely anything could happen at 30,000 feet! I felt much more secure right where I was.

Denise: His surgery had not been scheduled yet. The hospital was waiting to hear from the insurance company. The plan was to air ambulance him back to Vancouver until the cardiologist got on the phone and told them his patient could not be moved. He needed to have the surgery now!

Jim and Paula followed me to the car rental and waited while I returned the car, helped me with the bags and Paula got a special pass to go through security and walk me to the gate.

When I arrived back in Honolulu I went to the hotel that the nurse had suggested but I didn't like it. I didn't feel safe there. So, with our entire luggage (two garment bags, three suitcases and two carry-ons) I moved to the Ala Moana Hotel right at the Ala Moana Shopping Center. I then went directly to the hospital to be with Steve. He looked great! I was exhausted!

It's a Go!

On Sunday, I was told that authorization to proceed with the operation had been received the day before but the OR did not operate on the weekends. I was scheduled for surgery on Monday. I was surprisingly calm waiting for Monday. My thinking was as follows: First, I could not be in better hands or in a better place with Dr. Grattan and Dr. Kai and the Straub Medical Center. Second, everything was now out of my control so there was absolutely no sense worrying about it. What would be would be! Third, as a psychologist I knew that the best thing I could do was to be positive and confident. I held onto the belief that I would be fine. Finally, what I found happening was I became an observer in the process. I really detached emotionally from it.

Armed with this perspective, I approached the first life-threatening event in my life. A concluding thought about the necessity of having medical travel insurance. If I were to have had this adventure without the insurance, it would have been a near "bankruptcy event", the total costs running well into six figures!

Denise: I was so thankful that Steve was receiving excellent care. We were told that Dr. Grattan was one of the five top thoracic surgeons in the US. I was also relieved that Steve would not be air-lifted to Vancouver because what if something happened flying over the Pacific. There is nowhere to land!

Monday Afternoon and it's off to the OR

The first concrete indication that it was actually going to happen was the visit from the nurse's aide to shave me, not quite from head to toe, but almost!

The operation was scheduled for 1:30 p.m. and about 45 minutes before, I was transferred to the OR. Denise stayed with me as long as she was allowed and kissed me and said that she would see me in recovery.

My recollection of the events that followed are at best sketchy. I can remember being placed in the hall outside the OR and being visited by a variety of nurses and doctors who each verified my identity. We wouldn't want to be operating on the wrong patient now, would we? I was then wheeled into the OR and transferred to the operating table. The anesthetic was administered, and that's all I remember.

When I regained consciousness, I was in the ICU. I must have breathed a sigh of relief at coming through the procedure successfully, but I was not aware of it. I was fairly uncomfortable, with a tube down my throat and two tubes draining my abdominal cavity. The nurse told me that the next step forward would be to have the breathing tube removed.

My assumption is that everything went according to plan as the breathing tube was removed, and I gradually became more and more clear headed. When it came time for my first solid food, Jell-O, the nurse began to feed me at which point I said that I could feed myself. She later commented that she had never seen a patient be able to do that so soon after the procedure. This was another small indication of my overall good health.

Denise: Just before Steve went into the OR, Dr. Grattan came over and introduced himself. I asked him when Steve would be in recovery. He replied, "Come back around 4:00 p.m." His demeanor inspired confidence. I turned, kissed Steve and told him I'd see him later. The best thing now for me was to return to my hotel room for a nap.

An hour or so later, I showered and returned to the hospital. It was close to 7:00 p.m. when I finally had the chance to talk to Dr. Grattan. He told me he was pleased with the surgery, and I could visit Steve in the ICU. I went in to see him. He was sleeping with a breathing tube and not conscious. I whispered in his ear, "I love you, and I'll see you later." Then I phoned our friends Nancy and Mickey for a ride back to the hotel.

Tuesday Afternoon and it's back to the Ward from the ICU

By early Tuesday afternoon, I was transferred back to the ward. My memories of this process are quite spotty. All I can recall is feeling relieved to have made it "through the gauntlet" and comforted that I was back in familiar surroundings with familiar, friendly faces. The staff commented on how well I looked after the procedure.

I was encumbered now with drainage tubes and IV drips, which made moving around a bit challenging. I settled in on the first leg of my road to recovery. During this time, I was quite bored but did not have the will or energy to do anything. At this point, I wish that I had kept a journal, but at the time, I had no interest in doing that either. I know that I had many thoughts and feelings but unfortunately, they are all gone now.

Denise: I was told that I could visit Steve Tuesday afternoon when he was back in the ward, so the next morning I went for an hour massage. As a person who deals with chronic pain, I had to look after myself, and it would also help me relax.

Tuesday Afternoon to Sunday Afternoon - Recovery

I was impressed by how quickly they wanted to get me moving. The second day the nurses had me sitting up in my reclining chair for my meals. I also walked to the bathroom rather than using a bed pan. However, I still used the portable urinal since they were tracking my intake and outflow of fluids. The amount of discharge from my draining tubes was also measured regularly.

The final requirement for me to leave the hospital was to be able to walk 1,200 steps, so I was urged to get started on that agenda as soon as possible. Richard, one of the nurses' aides, and I would walk up and down the hallway, starting at 300 steps. I added 300 steps a day until I reached 1,200, which occurred on Saturday.

During my recovery, I was initially visited regularly by Drs. Grattan and Kai. However, as it was evident that I was mending quite quickly, I saw them less frequently. I also had some interactions with the endocrinologist, Dr. Leonard Kryston who also played a central role in the "supplement drama", which I will discuss later.

At one point, my blood sugar levels were elevated so that was being monitored as well.

Although I have many stories concerning my interactions with the staff, I will share my favorite. I was attended to by a nurses' aide whom I only saw a few times. We got talking about what happened to me, which prompted her to share that her favorite part of the operation was the saw! I very quickly told her that was way too much information, and I did not want to hear any more.

There are a lot of complaints about hospital food. However, I must admit that I found the food just fine. I think that I was so grateful to be safe, and cared for, not to mention hungry, the food simply was not an issue! My recovery proceeded quickly and without event. The hospital had no interest in keeping me any longer than was absolutely necessary. So, when I was ready, I was sent on my way.

Denise: While Steve was recovering, I established a routine of visiting him, which included either taking a taxi or walking to or from the hotel and Straub. In terms of food, I would either get a meal from the hospital cafeteria and eat with Steve in his room or go back to the Ala Moana Shopping Center and dine alone in one of the many restaurants. On one occasion, I noted how surreal it was sitting and looking out at the ocean having dinner and thinking, "My husband is in the hospital recovering from surgery, and I'm here!"

Sunday Afternoon – I'm Discharged and it's off to the Ala Moana Hotel!

When Denise returned from Maui, she checked into a hotel that was recommended by one of the nurses. However, it was not suitable so she relocated to the Ala Moana where we had stayed on several occasions. It was within walking distance to the hospital and attached to the Ala Moana Shopping Center! Need I say more!

Richard offered to assist us in transferring to the hotel so mid-afternoon we packed up my belongings and took a taxi to the Ala Moana. It was great having Richard along since all the carrying was looked after.

The change from a controlled to an uncontrolled environment was tiring. I was only interested in getting into bed! My next target was meetings with my two doctors on Wednesday morning to see if I would be given clearance to travel.

Denise: I remember being so exhausted, and my anxiety gave me chest pains. One evening when I was visiting Steve, Dr. Grattan suggested I go to Emergency to get checked out. I was fine. One cardiac event was enough for this trip!

It was wonderful to have Steve back at the hotel with me. As he settled in, Richard stayed while I went to Long's Drugs to pick up Steve's prescriptions and buy lunch for the three of us.

My Honolulu Convalescence

Our initial thought was that recuperating in the hotel would almost be like a holiday and we even talked about extending our stay in Honolulu for a week since I had made arrangements to have all my commitments covered. However, a hotel room, even if it is in Honolulu, is still a hotel room, and we quite quickly found the space confining. The travel insurance company also had no interest in subsidizing our stay in Hawaii a moment longer than necessary!

Richard came by on Tuesday to give Denise a break. She did not want to leave me alone and frankly, I did not want to be left alone either. So while Denise was out and about, Richard walked with me and saw that I was taken care of. This arrangement worked fine until Denise returned and if you think the room was too small for two, it was definitely way too small for three!

My time was spent walking up and down the hallway, watching television, and resting. I still did not have the energy or will to read but I did write my one and only diary entry. It read:

Tuesday – 2:07 p.m.

Here we are, sitting on the lanai of our room on the twentieth floor of the Ala Moana Hotel. There is a gentle, warm breeze, a partially cloudy sky, with the green hills in the distance.

In a past life (before my operation, which I would come to learn is referred to as CABG [pronounced "cabbage" meaning coronary artery bypass graft]) we would probably be off to walk the Mall or go down to Waikiki and stroll along the beach.

Since I had already taken a 24-minute round trip to the bank to refinance our little adventure, more rest and relaxation will be the order of the day with another short walk in the evening to get my 30 minutes.

And that's it! If I could turn back the clock, the one thing that I would definitely have done is to have a tape recorder and dictate my ongoing thoughts. Unfortunately, the nuances have been lost.

Denise: I really just wanted to sleep but I thought it best to take a break and let Richard look after Steve. I had not seen Waikiki for a while so I hopped on a tourist tram and toured the city for a few hours. It was a relaxing diversion.

I Get Clearance to Fly!

Wednesday morning, we took a taxi to Straub to see the surgeon and cardiologist. We met with Dr. Grattan and then Dr. Kai. Dr. Grattan was pleased with my progress and said he saw no reason to prevent us from flying home as soon as we could arrange a flight. Dr. Kai concurred. After securing documentation for the airline that stated I was not a risk to fly, we left the hospital, thankful for that chapter being closed. To celebrate, we went to the Honolulu Academy of Art for lunch. Our friend Nancy is a volunteer there, and it is one of our favourite places to visit whenever we are in Honolulu.

A Visit from Emily

As I mentioned, Emily lives on the Big Island and when she heard about what happened to me, she was eager to help in any way she could. We told her that while I was in the hospital, there was very little she could do so we were successful in discouraging her from visiting. You must understand that when Emily decides to do something, it gets done, and she decided that she was coming to help and be supportive in any way she could.

She arrived the Wednesday afternoon and met us at the hotel. Emily had "wheels" so we were able to take care of some errands. It was off to Long's Drugs to sort out some medications and buy the packaging material to return some supplements* to *Alive and Well* in Maui. (* My supplements are an adventure in themselves and will be addressed later.)

After all this activity, I was not up to going out for dinner so Emily volunteered to get takeout and brought back a terrific Japanese meal, which conformed with my dietary restrictions. Emily left the food with us to go and have dinner with her mother, and Denise and I had a picnic in the room. It was wonderful to see Emily and touching to know that she would go to all the trouble and expense that she did to be with us. True friends are to be cherished.

On Thursday, it was off to *Down to Earth* in search of Macadamia nut oil without success and *Bragg's*, a substitute for soy sauce, which is very high in sodium. This search was successful. Then it was off to lunch at *The House Without a Key* at the Halekulani Hotel in Waikiki, our absolutely favorite place in Honolulu. Emily insisted on treating. It was then back to the hotel with Emily bidding us farewell and a safe trip home.

The balance of the day was spent packing and wondering how we would ever fit everything into our suitcases. Thursday was quite a social day in that for dinner we met Nancy and Mickey for dinner in the restaurant at the top of the hotel.

Denise: For me, it was comforting to be with Emily. Our day with her was so special, and I'll never forget my lunch at the Halekulani: seafood salad and a glass of Chardonnay!

Friday Afternoon – We Fly Home!

Friday morning was consumed with finishing packing. We had called Richard to help us vacate the hotel and get us to the airport. Once again, it was great to have him there to help us. It's amazing how I took things like lifting suitcases for granted. I was beginning to appreciate how limited I was going to be over the next few months.

Richard had ordered up a limo since we knew that we would not be able to fit our luggage into a regular taxi. Now it was off to the airport. We were hoping that Richard would be able to accompany us right to the gate but unfortunately, that was not to be. We were flying on WestJet, and they said they would get us to the gate.

Richard waited while we checked in; having the documentation from the hospital proved to be essential. We were thankful that we took the time to secure the letters. We said our goodbyes to Richard and proceeded through security.

We were met by a WestJet staff member with a cart and were transferred in style to the gate. We were approached by the captain, who was quite concerned about me and wanted to know my condition and that I was cleared to fly. The conversation was completely out of character with all my other flying experiences; members of the flight crew have never taken any interest in me before!

We boarded the plane, which was not full and had excellent seats at the front. The flight home was uneventful, with the flight crew being attentive and concerned. I breathed a giant sigh of relief as we landed in Vancouver. I made it home!

Denise: As Steve said, our flight home was uneventful. Thanks again WestJet. Yes, a big sigh of relief to be back home and after clearing Customs, we were met by Steve's cousin and nephew. I had been carrying such an emotional "load" and seeing them, I finally broke down and cried. Our support system had arrived! Through it all I never felt like I needed a family member to fly to Hawaii to help us. I knew deep down I could do whatever I needed to do.

Part 3

Convalescing at Home and Beyond

It's Good to Be Home!

We both breathed a huge sigh of relief when we landed safely in Vancouver. We made it! My nephew Jon and my cousin Gary volunteered to pick us up at the airport and take us home. The first adjustment was becoming accustomed to being somewhat limited in what I could do. "No heavy lifting", which for all intent and purpose translated into "no lifting", became the order of the day and this new rule was immediately confronted by the task of getting the luggage into the house. Thanks Jon and Gary! After the usual unpacking of essentials, I settled into bed, overwhelmed by the feeling of being grateful to be home. The complete unpacking task took Denise two weeks! Remember, no lifting!

Settling into a Routine

Although the scope of my activities and energy were limited, I had this developing sense of freedom. My responsibilities were covered, and I had nothing to do but focus on getting well. With all of life's intrusions being held at bay, the traditional pressures associated with being at home vanished. I mused that this is what retirement might look like.

Our days were occupied with walking, grocery shopping, visiting the doctor, and relaxing. I had great plans to use the time to catch up on some writing projects and office organizing but unfortunately, I found it difficult to focus so the "down time" did not translate into what I would define as "productive time". I was amazed that the process of healing in itself was a full time job.

One of the takeaways from Straub was my Heart Hugger, which was a harness that replaced the traditional pillow and belt to be used in the event of a sneeze or cough. This protected the incision from experiencing any undue stress. An added benefit of the Heart Hugger was its use as a visual signal that something was different with me. When we were in crowds shopping or walking in the mall, people avoided bumping into me, which was very helpful. The Heart Hugger became a constant companion until I was given official permission that I did not need to use it any more.

Driving Mr. Stevie

Another takeaway from Straub were the guidelines concerning riding in a car. I was told not to drive for at least six weeks or until I was given clearance by my doctor. I was also told never to be a passenger in a seat that had an airbag. Evidently, an airbag event would be very nasty business for me as I was healing. It could even prove to be fatal! Even though the chances of it happening were very low, it made no sense to take this chance.

Denise became the designated driver, which was a new role for her that she reluctantly assumed since even at the best of times, she preferred not to drive. My car had a passenger seat airbag but Denise's did not and she liked her car anyway. Until I was told that I could resume driving, I had to become accustomed to being a passenger. As I became more and more active, my nephew Nick also helped out by driving me to my meetings. I resented the loss of my independence but quite enjoyed being a passenger, even if I had to ride in the back seat!

Following My New Dietary Guidelines

As was indicated in Part 1, I have always been interested in nutrition and conscious of my eating habits. In fact, I have written a book on nutrition, aptly titled *Nutritional Intelligence®: Eating for Life on the 80/20 Plan*. One of the premises of the book is that specific diets do not work very well, and the suggestion is for people to understand the consequences of their eating choices and assume responsibility for acquiring the knowledge for making intelligent choices.

Pareto's Principle or the "80/20 Rule" forms the basic guideline for the system. If you are behaving yourself and on the program 80 percent of the time, you can go off the program 20 percent of the time without serious consequences.

After getting my dietary marching orders in Hawaii, 80/20 quickly became 95/5! I had to watch my fat and sodium intake very closely but otherwise it was just being more vigilant with the guidelines that I was already following more or less. No more exceptions or transgressions now! I left for Hawaii at 205 pounds and returned at 190 pounds forty-seven days later. However, much to my delight, on the more rigorous program I continued to lose weight and currently sit at 177.5 at the end of May, 2009. I would be untruthful if I said that I didn't miss the old flexibility, but I have been able to make adjustments, which will be detailed later.

The "Episode"

I was naturally concerned about my heart and related issues so one of the things that I did was periodically monitor my pulse. The doctor had told me that the odd skipped heartbeat was normal but if it persisted, it could be a problem.

On the evening of February 20th, I was feeling a little off – palpitations and skipped heartbeats. The following morning, I was still not right so I called my doctor's office and went to their first come, first served Saturday clinic. The doctor on call took my blood pressure, and it was quite elevated. Since she did not have the facilities to do an EKG and not wanting to take any chances, she decided to send me to Emergency at the Vancouver General Hospital. This time an ambulance was not considered necessary!

The VGH ER Experience

We arrived at Emergency without event and went through the admissions process. I was put on a gurney, which was placed at station J in the hallway with an excellent view of all the action. This was to be my "home" for the next eight hours.

I was given the usual series of tests and procedures: blood samples were taken, and an EKG was administered and pulse and blood pressure were regularly monitored. The ER was busy but did not appear to be overwhelmed. However, I quickly made the assessment that I was low man on the totem pole in terms of need for treatment.

Denise and I spent the day in the hallway waiting for something to happen. The only comfort I had was the belief that, if there was something seriously wrong with me, I would be treated differently. I must be OK! In the early evening, I was moved to a separate examination area and visited by two of the residents from the Cardiac Care

Unit. At this point, the level of attention increased significantly. I was even provided with a tuna fish sandwich since I had not eaten all day. Finally, around 9:00 p.m., I was informed that they had found a bed for me in the Cardiac Care Unit, and I was being transferred there for observation. I met this news with very mixed feelings. I did not want to be in the hospital again. However, if I needed to be, then I was definitely in the right place. I reverted to my pre-operation mindset, affirming, with positive feelings, that what will be, will be.

The Cardiac Care Unit

The set-up in the unit was very similar to what I experienced in Hawaii. I was made comfortable and like before, knew that I was in really good hands. My nephew Jon and my cousin Gary arrived to keep me company, and Denise went home for a very well-earned rest.

I was informed that the cardiologist would see me the next day so all I could do was rest and have positive thoughts that all would be well. However, I could not help thinking that my concern in the morning might have been more a result of unwarranted worry and not a legitimate problem because, at the moment, I felt just fine!

Denise: It was traumatic for me sitting there, Steve lying on a stretcher in the corridor and watching car accident victims arrive on gurneys from ambulances. Then another wave brought several Vancouver City Police officers with a prisoner in handcuffs and shortly after a trucker was brought in. He was swearing and yelling in excruciating pain. Finally, he was wheeled into Acute Care.

I was numb. Feeling a touch on my shoulder and hearing a voice say, "It should be a bit quieter now," I looked up and saw to my surprise it was one of the police officers showing empathy and care in an otherwise chaotic environment. How kind he was to us.

Soon after, the doctor arrived and Steve was eventually moved to the Cardiac Care Unit. I knew again that he was in very good hands and that it was time for me to go home and sleep. Gary would take over for a while.

A Fortuitous Meeting with the Cardiologist

Sunday morning, the cardiologist and residents made their rounds. I was told that Dr. Saul Isserow was on duty that weekend. "The" cardiologist became "My" cardiologist! Good fortune was smiling on me again. After a great deal of deliberation, Dr. Isserow was the name that I suggested to my doctor. Dr. Glanzberg was very familiar with him and referred me but my appointment with Saul was yet to be scheduled and could take at least three to six months. This visit to the hospital had now accomplished the impossible, an immediate meeting with Dr. Isserow! I was on the fast track! Any stress and inconvenience associated with my stay in the hospital immediately became a non-issue.

Adjusting My Meds and Related Benefits

I have met many doctors in my day but I have never experienced a doctor with a "bedside manner" like Dr. Isserow's. He was calming and reassuring and had a way of focusing and communicating that left no doubt in my mind that he was absolutely present and committed to me. I very quickly understood the reasons for his high demand.

He reviewed my test results and the documentation from my operation in Hawaii. A number of the my blood test scores on my liver panel were out of range, which was attributed to the high dose of Lipitor that I was on so I was taken off that medication until those readings returned to the normal range. In addition, the dose of my beta blocker was increased and an ACE inhibitor was added to my regimen. This is the second positive outcome from my hospital stay that would not have happened nearly as quickly otherwise.

The third outcome was the reassurance from Dr. Isserow that there was nothing wrong with my heart, that the procedure was successful and that I should continue my recovery with the comfort in knowing that I was all right. He scheduled an echocardiogram and a stress test for me in early April prior to my appointment with him on April 20th. Mission accomplished!

Denise: I was also greatly impressed with Dr. Isserow's care and grateful that Steve was now "on track" with his cardiologist.

Highlights and Overall Impressions

I now had experiences in two emergency rooms and two cardiac care units. I received much quicker treatment at Maui Memorial Emergency than I did at Vancouver General but it really is not a fair comparison, the latter being much busier. In terms of the cardiac units, I was very pleasantly surprised. The care I received in Vancouver was absolutely comparable to what I experienced at the Straub Center in Honolulu. The nurses were competent and friendly, and the care I received was outstanding. Any comments about the substandard nature of our health care system bandied about in the press was certainly not substantiated by my experience. Waiting for treatment is one thing, but once you are in the system, you are well cared for.

Post "Episode" Recovery

I returned home relieved and with as clean a bill of health as I could reasonably expect. We settled back into our routine, which involved walking, shopping, cooking, napping, and watching some TV. I was still wearing my Heart Hugger and not driving so my movements were restricted. Any thoughts of returning to work were quickly dispelled since I simply did not have the energy. However, by the end of February, I felt strong enough to attend the morning session of one of my groups but I was pretty much "done" by noon so I was well aware that I had a long way to go if I was to convene my groups in March. Unfortunately, I still did not have the energy or interest to begin writing. That agenda would have to wait.

A Stress Test and Echocardiogram

In preparation for my appointment with Dr. Isserow, I had to have an echocardiogram and take a stress test. I was quite apprehensive about the stress test, wondering how long I would be able to last and whether it would reveal problems of which I was unaware. Both the echocardiogram and stress test experience proceeded without event. I was able to last nine minutes on the treadmill with my pulse and blood pressure returning to normal levels within the appropriate time frame. Now all I had to do was wait for my appointment on April 20th.

My Meeting with Dr. Isserow

Denise and I arrived at the appointed hour. I did not think about it at the time, but this would be the last occasion when I was chauffeured.

I was given the "green light" to drive, have a bath, abandon my Heart Hugger and generally resume normal activities. I could even play golf! We were told that the success of a bypass procedure was determined by four factors, the first three being technical with the last one being lifestyle. The first three factors were the quality of the receptor sites, the quality of the grafting material and the health of the heart. Saul said that I was done in by my genetics; there was probably nothing that I could have done to prevent what happened to me. In fact, my clean lifestyle probably delayed the occurrence of the event and lessened its severity. But the highlight of the visit was feedback on the results of my stress test. The last time I took the test was about four years ago, and I was able to last six minutes. This time, after not exercising for three and a half months, I managed nine minutes, a 50 percent improvement! This was truly good news. It's an open question as to how long and to what extent my condition had been impeding me to perform at an optimum level in a wide variety of activities.

We also spent some time talking about my supplementation regime. I was told that I could resume taking my supplements but that it was probably not necessary to take quite so many. Dr. Kai would agree. The next task was to see a specialist to sort this all out. Since some of the items on my liver panel were still slightly out of range, the decision to put me back on a statin was further delayed.

Finally, Dr. Isserow had a few comments on my diet. He was basically satisfied that I knew what to do. However, he did make two specific suggestions: completely eliminate butter and consume only one egg yolk per week. I was ready for no butter but not one egg yolk! These two restrictions effectively eliminated all commercially baked goods. The net result of this change was the total elimination of all high calorie, low nutritional value foods from my diet.

Dr. Isserow reassured me that I was just fine and my healing and recovery were proceeding very well. He told me to resume my full range of activities but cautioned me that the driver should not be the first club that I took out of the bag! We were sent to his receptionist to book my follow-up, which was to be on October 19th preceded by another stress test. I was through the gate!

Push-ups, Power Walking and Workouts with Light Hand Weights

The first part of my old regimen that I reinstated was pushups. For a number of years, every morning I would see how many pushups I could do. I was told that they were not "real" pushups since I did not fully extend my arms and relied a great deal on momentum. My best effort was ninety-three! Keep in mind that this was with my coronary artery problems. This time I made the decision to do real pushups. I started with one every morning and added one each week. Currently, I am at eight with lots of reserve. It will be interesting to see how high I can go.

The second part of our old regimen is fast walking. We have a route through a park near our house that takes us 30 minutes if we walk quite briskly. Our best time to date is $27\frac{1}{4}$ minutes, which is moving right along. My goal is to walk 10,000 steps a day. I have also begun walking at home using light hand weights. I've started with one pounders and every six weeks I'll add a pound.

Resolving the Supplementation Question

A few years ago, I had my doctor refer me to a MD who specialized in supplementation. He reviewed my list and for the most part thought that what I was taking was all right, although he did comment that the value of some of the items was questionable, labeling them as "marketing". My major concern was the potential interaction of my supplements with my medications, a situation that I never had to deal with before.

While in the hospital in Hawaii, I was taken off of all my supplements but was interested in observing that part of my daily meds were a multivitamin and folic acid. Dr. Kryston, the endocrinologist did review my list and made several observations: anything that might interfere with the statin, Lipitor, had to be stopped. This included grapefruit pectin and red rice yeast. Since I was put on a daily Aspirin, Provex CV, a grape skin, grapeseed product also had to be stopped since it had some of the same effects as the Aspirin. My efforts to have this issue resolved in Hawaii were unsuccessful, and I was told that my cardiologist in Vancouver would be the one to sort it out. Dr. Grattan's position on supplementation was that it was unnecessary and for some supplements, potentially harmful. Dr. Kai's comment to me was that I was probably taking too many supplements. Dr. Isserow's position was that he did not see any problem with taking the supplements although he did not see that there was any clear medical benefit to doing so for most of them. The doctors in Hawaii would concur. He left the decision up to me and the specialist. We pared down my list and this process continues to be a work in progress. More on this in a few pages.

Resolving the "Travel Insurance" Question – Part 1

One of the questions that popped into my mind was "How can I travel with insurance coverage if I have a 'prior condition'?" I knew that there must be lots of people that have undergone bypass surgery that are traveling. So, how does that happen? After making a call to the insurance company, I was referred to the relevant pages in the agreement. A prior condition is covered if you are considered "stable". Stable was defined by my insurer as not having any reoccurrence or any problems related to the condition for 90 days prior to departure. This includes changes to any medications in terms of dosages, either increases or decreases, and additions of different medications and/or deletions from your current regimen.

Since I was scheduled for my follow-up session with Dr. Isserow in October, our holiday plans in December were in jeopardy. I called his office, explained my dilemma, and requested that he see me in late August. She called back and countered with mid-January. I commented that Dr. Isserow did not seem too concerned about me – in a good way! She agreed. So here I am on June 11, 2009, healing in process, with my doctor comfortable with my progress.

Resolving the "Travel Insurance" Question – Part 2

The more important question concerning travel insurance was the status of my claim for Hawaii. Since our return, I had received numerous invoices from a variety of the health care providers requesting payment for their services. As instructed, I forwarded all of them to the medical travel insurance company. There was also some confusion concerning their receipt of the appropriate records from my family doctor. As a part of the claims process, we also submitted all of our out-of-pocket living expenses for our time in Honolulu.

As time passed, we heard nothing, and this uncertainty was a concern. At last, on Wednesday, June 10th, a cheque arrived covering all of our out-of-pocket expenses so it appears that this chapter of the saga is also coming to a favorable conclusion!

Dealing with the "Sludge"!

One of the results of the ultrasound, which was performed on my internal organs as a final procedure before I was discharged from the Vancouver General Hospital in February, was the discovery of "sludge" in my gallbladder. I came to learn that there are three types of people, those who produce gall stones, those who produce sludge, which consists of the same material as gall stones, but for some reason, does not form them, and those who have neither.

The specialist prescribed some medication and also mentioned that drinking lemon juice would be helpful. After I completed this regimen, try as I might, I could not convince any of my doctors to order a follow-up ultrasound on my gallbladder. They were simply not concerned and were not willing to spend medical resources on me for this purpose.

Through all this, no one could tell me how I developed this condition so it was off to the Internet. I very quickly discovered that one of the causes of gallbladder sludge was rapid weight loss. I definitely qualified! Mystery solved.

Supplementation Revisited!

I am a member of a Psychology Discussion Group, which is a part of my continuing education requirement. In one of our sessions, a physician specializing in integrative medicine was recommended as a resource for addressing my gallbladder concerns as well as possibly shedding some more light on my quest to resolve the supplementation question.

I secured a referral from Dr. Glanzberg and met Dr. G. B. Ryder. He is a medical doctor as well as a pharmacologist and uses VEGA Testing as a part of his practice. The VEGA testing process is based on functional spectroscopy, which measures the body's response to various substances. He identified that there was a problem with my gallbladder and successfully addressed it. I felt better.

The next step was to review all my supplements. He tested their suitability for me with surprising results. He found that the majority of the supplements that I was taking were toxic or harmful for me. A second smaller group was neutral; they did no harm but also provided no benefit. The third much smaller group was beneficial. The outcome of this process was that my status as a poster boy for taking supplements was at an end!

My current regimen consists of my meds plus folic acid, saw palmetto, omega 3 fish oil, vitamin D drops and N-Acetyl L Cysteine. Dr. Isserow subsequently removed the folic acid. Even my whey protein powder, which was the centerpiece of my daily protein shake, failed to make the cut. It was replaced by a rice-based protein product that also includes a comprehensive multivitamin/mineral. My doctors in Hawaii would approve! (Complete lists and recipes are included in the Appendix.)

As a further comment on the use of supplementation, a handout from Dr. Ryder provides some useful information. It is included in Appendix D.

My First Disciple!

The news of my experience spread fairly quickly through my circle of friends and acquaintances with varying responses. One friend took my experience as a giant wake-up call and took immediate action to get himself checked out. He was referred to, of all people, Dr. Saul Isserow, who ran some tests and in fact discovered that he did indeed have a problem! My dear friend then launched into a revision of his eating and drinking habits resulting in the loss of forty pounds!

When we had lunch at the end of November, which was our first opportunity to see each other, he credited me with giving him the inspiration and motivation to change his ways and potentially, save him from a heart "event" with unknown but possibly fatal consequences.

At lunch, I ordered a salad with all of my usual caveats. His response was, "Make that two!"

Beyond Convalescing – Maintaining the "Status Quo!

Within the constant backdrop of the knowledge that my life had changed dramatically and would never return to the way it was, we were nevertheless, very much back to our usual routine. My energy had returned, and we were looking forward to returning to Maui.

$\mathcal{P}art$ 4

Returning to "The Scene of the Crime!"

Feelings and Greetings

We both approached our holiday with a mixture of excitement and anxiety, excitement because we were getting away for a well-deserved rest after a very stressful year and anxiety because of the events earlier this year and the nagging fear that there was another "shoe" lurking that might drop!

The flight was uneventful, and we slipped seamlessly into our usual routine. When we arrived at "The Cove", we were greeted by Su, the Office Manager who, over the years has become a good friend. She hugged us both and made us feel like we had truly arrived at our home away from home. Greg, the new Resident Manager, helped us with the luggage, and we began the process of settling in. We both looked at each other and breathed a sigh of relief. Denise cried. We had made it back successfully!

Denise: I felt like I had been holding my breath for the past year in anticipation of something else happening. Being back truly meant we had made it!

Closing the Loop on a Phone Conversation

When I was in the hospital, one of the calls I received was from a friend from Vancouver who stopped by the condo on Maui to say hi. One of the owners saw him looking lost and asked if he needed any help. He stated that he was looking for us and when Pat told him what had happened, she thought that he was going to have an "event" as well. He just looked at her in disbelief claiming that it just could not be.

When I talked to Bob from the hospital, he told me how shocked he was but having Pat describe his reactions that revealed the extent of his surprise and disbelief added another dimension. It's comforting to know that we were missed and cared about.

Settling In

As Jerry Seinfeld in *Seinfeld* had claimed it was a show about nothing, we have a holiday routine about nothing as well. As was mentioned, we have breakfast, nap, read, shop for groceries (a major activity), walk, which includes looking for golf balls, cook dinner and watch TV. Denise and I also use the time to write.

It never ceases to amaze me that over twenty years, we have not tired of this routine. We do not sunbathe and frequent the beach only on rare occasions! The two major differences this year are: (1) going out to restaurants is much less attractive as an activity since I hold to my requirements for plain food quite vigorously. Serving up food devoid of butter, egg yolks and salt gets to be a bit of a bore for both me and the servers! The bottom line is we cook food that meets our needs better than the expensive restaurants.

The second difference for me is a heightened awareness of how I am feeling. Almost every day, when I would have a slight pain or some indigestion, I would immediately begin to worry about myself. When this would happen I consciously would remind myself that I got completely checked out by Dr. Isserow before we left, and he gave me the "green light". He did not have any concerns about me traveling, so why should I?

Reuniting with Mel

Mel, the Resident Manager's wife, was one of the "angels" who appeared to help Denise when she came back to Maui to close up our unit. She graciously offered to help Denise pack and volunteered to stay with her overnight in the unit. This was of great assistance and comfort for Denise. We had been looking for Mel and finally ran into her in the parking lot. She was delighted to see us, and we both thanked her again for all her help last January. She told us she would drop by 202 (our unit) for a visit before we left.

A Meeting with Dr. Ben Azman

One of my agendas for our return to Hawaii was to thank all the doctors personally for their care last January. I had made arrangements to see Drs. Kai and Grattan from home and planned to make the calls to the doctors on Maui after we arrived. I was looking forward to seeing them but, as I was to discover, the process was far more complex than I initially anticipated.

I called the West Maui Clinic and was able after some effort, to explain that I just wanted to stop by and see Dr. Azman to thank him, and not to have a "formal" appointment. That part of the process went quite smoothly. However, as the time approached for the actual visit, Denise became increasingly anxious about it. She wanted to go with me, but she was not sure whether she would come in with me.

On December 23rd, we drove to the West Maui Clinic and the closer we got, the more anxious Denise became, and as we arrived, she said she simply could not go in. The whole experience came flooding back to her.

I went into the office, and the receptionist told me that Dr. Azman would be with me shortly. We greeted each other, and I thanked him for the excellent care he had provided for me and credited him with saving my life. I told him that I was writing a book about my experiences and invited him to contribute to the foreword. He was very appreciative that I made the effort to come and thank him and honored to be asked to contribute. He gave me his e-mail address, we said goodbye, and I went looking for Denise. However, after our meeting, I felt quite unsettled. What Denise felt in anticipation of the visit, I experienced after the fact. This feeling was to stay with me for the next several days and intensified as I made arrangements to see Drs. Massenburg and Dr. Gordon. Evidently, I too was harboring all kinds of feelings related to my "adventures".

A Meeting with Dr. Ben Massenburg

In our telephone conversation, we sorted out when he would be at the hospital. He told me that he would be available to see me depending upon work demands, during those times. Late morning on Saturday, January 2nd we drove "on our own steam" to Kahului to the Maui Memorial Hospital. I did not know what to expect and was thinking that he would appear and that we would have a brief interaction in the Emergency waiting room. We parked and went into Emergency. I of course never saw it from this perspective so it looked totally unfamiliar to me. We asked an attending receptionist if he was available and she went about finding him for us.

After about 15–20 minutes, he appeared and ushered us into a private waiting room. I thanked him again for all his help, and he expressed his appreciation for taking the time to come in to see him. He commented that the emergency physicians rarely find out what happens to the people that they see after they are discharged. I had written him a thank you letter to which he did not respond so I made the assumption that it was not important to him. That assumption couldn't have been more wrong!

When he saw me a year ago, he was cool and very businesslike. Consequently, I was pleasantly surprised when, after telling me how good I looked, he gave me a big hug! What a wonderful validation! We talked for about half an hour. He also accepted the invitation to contribute to the book's foreword and provided me with his contact information. My meeting with Dr. Massenburg far exceeded any expectations that I had for our encounter.

Dinner with the Greens

This year, when Paula and Jim Green arrived, we invited them to dinner at one of the local restaurants to thank them again for their kindness, generosity, and help when we were dealing with my emergency situation last year. Having them help Denise return the rental car and drive her to the airport provided a tremendous amount of support for her. It was gratifying to have an opportunity to sit down and tell them how much their assistance mattered to us.

A Meeting with Dr. Pamela Gordon

Dr. Gordon was the last doctor on Maui. We stopped by her office, which was located in the Kaiser Permanente Complex in Kahului. She remembered me and like Dr. Massenburg, was delighted that I took the time to stop by and see her. I guess my behavior was really quite different than the norm. She was pleased to see that I was doing well and also agreed to contribute to the foreword of the book. With this meeting, the loop was closed on my Maui medical team.

A Visit from Emily

We convinced Emily to accept our gift of a "fully funded" day trip to Maui. We picked her up at the airport and went "up country" to the General Store in Hali'male, which is one of the premier restaurants on Maui, located amongst the sugarcane fields on the slopes of Haleakala in a renovated general store.

After lunch, we took a short drive down the road to introduce Emily to the Hui No'eau Visual Arts Center, which is a gallery and studio housed in one of the Baldwin family's estates. They were one of the original missionary families. It's one of our favorite places and Emily was delighted.

Here's a letter we received from Emily after her visit:

Dear Denise and Steve,

Thank you so much for a wonderful day! I loved every minute of it, from my flight over and back, seeing you drive up to the curb, to our terrific lunch at the General Store, and then over to the Baldwin Estate. It was super to see both of you healthy and happy, and especially after the events of last year, to be able to celebrate our friendship in such a positive space – both literally and figuratively.

I was very happy to finally get to the General Store, and the whole atmosphere was wonderful, light and great to share together!

I took some pictures documenting the trip over and our shots outside of the General Store, and hope that you like them.

Matt said that he knows Maui fairly well, but hadn't been to the Baldwin House either. It was so neat for you to introduce me to a unique and creative place, and I enjoyed walking around enjoying the pastoral scene.

When I got back home, Matt was still working on the framing for the wall base (footer). But, as I told him about the big waves, we drove down to the ocean (with Speed), and loved watching the sunset with those big waves. Speed was having the time of his life sniffing out all the scents down ocean way, and being thrilled to be part of our company. He and I have had parallel experiences today. (Unfortunately, Speed died in June of 2019.)

Look forward to seeing you in 2010 – you never know, I may be pulling up in front of your place with my new vehicle this year.

Enjoy your remaining time on Maui and have a smooth transition to Oahu and home.

Part 5

One Year Later

What a Difference a Year Makes!
January 8th

What a difference a year can make! Last year, this day marked the beginning of my "adventure". It started with the persistent indigestion and the rest, as they say, is history.

Although I did not sleep very well, probably in anticipation of the anniversary, today was what I hoped the eighth last year would have looked like! We ran a few errands, celebrated by buying Denise a lovely glass bead bracelet, walked through the pines, and brought in one of our favorite dinners. It was another beautiful day, and we walked 11,000 steps.

January 9th

This day last year, started with me having my angiogram, receiving the news, then waiting for clearance from the medical insurance company and preparing myself emotionally for the ordeal that I was about to experience. For Denise, it was providing me with emotional support and then heading off to Maui to pack up our unit.

This year, the day was spent leisurely packing up, running a few last minute errands and taking our final walk through the pines. However, I still felt quite unsettled and had to keep reassuring myself that it was a year later, and I was fine.

January 10th – Back To Honolulu

Last year this was a waiting day for me. This year, it was a traveling day for both of us. The trip went uneventfully; we checked into our hotel and then went to our favorite restaurant, *The House Without a Key* at the Halekulani, one of the high end hotels on Waikiki Beach for a celebration dinner. We made it!

January 11th

Last year, this was the day before my surgery. This year, it was Denise's turn! She needed to find an ophthalmologist to look at the corneal abrasion in her left eye, which was still bothering her. One way or another, we simply could not avoid visiting doctors. The afternoon was spent shopping, and in the evening we reunited with our friends Nancy and Mickey. In balance, it was a lovely day!

January 12th – My Anniversary Meetings
Dr. Wesley Kai

Today was the anniversary of my surgery. The major reason for returning to Honolulu was to visit Straub and thank all the people who provided me with such excellent care. My first appointment was with Dr. Kai. I initially expected to just have the opportunity to thank him but as events unfolded, the nurse weighed me and then led me into an examination room and took my blood pressure. Before I had a chance to say anything, I realized that my time with him was to be an "official" appointment. However, what started out to be an exercise in "closing the loop", very quickly became "high drama" when the nurse told me my blood pressure which from my perspective, was off the chart! Since April, my blood pressure had been fluctuating in the 115–125 over 70–80 range. This morning it was 150/96. *Yikes!* This information catapulted me into a very nasty place. I knew that I was apprehensive, but I never imagined that I was that apprehensive. The several minutes waiting for Dr. Kai to come into the examining room felt like an eternity.

Dr. Kai appeared, and I thanked him again for the role he played in saving my life. He then asked me how I was doing and updated his knowledge of my status since last January. He examined how my incision was healing, listened to my heart and retook my blood pressure, which he said had dropped. He did not seem concerned, so I decided that I would not be concerned either!

The bottom line was he was delighted with my progress and encouraged me to just keep up what I had been doing. We both thanked him again, and it was off to the next appointment.

Denise: When the nurse took Steve's blood pressure before Dr. Kai came in and it was higher than it has been for months, I tried not to show it. However, deep down I was "freaking out", saying to myself, "Oh God! Now what are we in for!" but I tried to maintain an outward calm to reassure Steve. I was so relieved when Dr. Kai retook his blood pressure and it had come down and I was so very glad when he told Steve, "You're doing super."

Dr. Leonard Kryston

When I arrived at Dr. Kryston's office, I spoke to the receptionist. I explained my request and fortunately he was in. He came to the reception window. He smiled, shook my hand and was delighted to accept my invitation to contribute to the book's foreword. Another successful encounter!

A Visit to the Ward

Next stop – 3 West! The nursing staff remembered me and were pleasantly surprised to receive the box of See's Chocolates that Denise and I brought for them. It was a three pounder! They seemed touched that we would take the time to stop by and thank them. My overriding impression upon returning to the ward was that it was a much smaller place than what I remembered. This was especially true of the long hallway that I had to walk up and down in preparation for my discharge. The hallway was much, much shorter than it was a year ago. So much for the reliability of perceptions and impressions.

Phil Odle

Part of my ward experience was my interactions with the dietitian, so I was pleased to have the opportunity to connect with him as well. He came out of a class that he was conducting, and he was pleased to see my progress. He also agreed to make a contribution to the book's foreword. Mission accomplished!

Dr. Mark Grattan

Unfortunately, we were unable to meet with Dr. Grattan. He was in surgery and there was no opportunity to thank him face to face.

Lunch with Nancy at the Academy

Our friend Nancy volunteers in the gift shop at the Honolulu Academy of Arts. The academy also has a great restaurant that's a block away from the Straub Clinic. It's one of our traditional activities when we visit Honolulu.

It's always great to spend time with Nancy. She has an infectious laugh! It was turkey sandwiches all round, hold the butter and mayo on the side for me!

January 13th

This was a traveling day both years. Last year in the afternoon I "traveled" from the ICU back to my room on the ward. This year we got up around 7:00 a.m.; it was a glorious morning! We went for a forty-minute walk along the water on Waikiki. The balance of the morning was spent having breakfast – a rice protein shake for me and oat bran porridge for Denise, and packing at a leisurely pace in preparation for our trip to the airport. We both wished that we could spend a few more days in Honolulu but realized it was time to go home.

January 14th – Back to Vancouver

The flight home was uneventful, and we landed safely. We now both experienced a huge sigh of relief since we were both worried about how this return trip was going to turn out. Would we encounter more health problems? Would I be okay? We made it. I now looked forward to continuing the process of healing and recovery.

January 19th – My Visit with Dr. Isserow

Denise and I arrived for my appointment with me dressed appropriately for my stress test. I was a bit apprehensive about it since I was hoping that I would be able to improve on my performance from last April when I lasted nine minutes. I was shaved and hooked up to the monitoring wires and tested for my resting blood pressure and heart rate. I reached the nine-minute mark and still felt that I was able to continue. The only discomfort that I had was a very dry mouth. As the treadmill lurched into its next stage, I began to jog. I had one more minute in me and lasted ten minutes, a slight improvement but less than I was hoping for. However, my blood pressure quickly recovered to 110 over 70, which was excellent.

We then waited for Dr. Isserow. He was very pleased with my progress. I updated him with my visit to Dr. Kai. He reviewed the results of my blood tests and decided that he would not put me back on a statin until all my liver readings were normal. I would revisit this monthly with Dr. Glanzberg. He told me that he was not going to change my medications, which I had expected. I did complain about the cough resulting from the Ramipril, and he asked me if I could live with it. I said that I could so that was that! I also asked about my one egg yolk a week restriction and asked if that could be relaxed.

His response was, "Why would you want to do that?" So much for that dietary change.

Dr. Isserow reassured me that I was doing very well and that he did not want to see me again until March 7, 2011. I took that to mean I was fine and should not be worrying about myself. We left Saul's office with a sigh of relief and the feeling that we had cleared the final hurdle. I just had to believe that if there was anything at all that was wrong or that I should be aware of, I would have been told.

I also asked Dr. Isserow if he would contribute to the foreword of the book, and he said he would be delighted to do so.

January 23rd – The End and the Beginning

One year ago, we flew home from Honolulu so it seemed appropriate to end the story on the anniversary of our return. Life had returned to our normal routine. I had two TEC meetings on the previous Wednesday and Thursday and was looking forward to two more on Tuesday and Wednesday, the 26th and 27th. On the one hand, we were glad to be home but on the other, we really missed Hawaii and were planning when we could return!

My recuperation year had ended and life after the bypass had begun. I was feeling fine and started my new adventure at my 1970 weight. However, I was very sensitive to any new twinge or sensation so had to constantly reassure myself that if anything was amiss, I would have been told.

January 28th – My Meeting with
Dr. Monte Glanzberg

This was the first meeting of the year 2010 in my regular bi-monthly follow ups. Initially, the plan was to write the book based on my experiences to this point in time. However, after finding out that the real benchmark for a reliable assessment of the relative success of the procedure that I went through was five years, not one, I decided to postpone finishing the book for another four years.

Part 6

Differences after One Year; Some Things Have Definitely Changed!

A Heightened Sensitivity to How I am Feeling

I have always been a bit of a hypochondriac, worrying about the implications of any new pain or sensation. However, now I have some very real concerns to attach to the "worrying". In spite of the reassurances from all my doctors, a twinge in my arm or chest sets off the alarm bells in a way that it did not before my "event". One of my challenges moving forward will be to remain calm and not upset myself or Denise when a perceived symptom appears.

Graciously Accepting Assistance

Upon our arrival at Honokeana Cove in December, 2009, the first task after all the greetings was to find Greg, the new Resident Manager, and ask him if he could help us transfer our luggage to the unit. I simply had to get over linking moving our bags by myself with my image of self-sufficiency. I am delighted to report that I am now totally comfortable graciously accepting this type of assistance.

One of my pet peeves is to be asked at the check-out counter at the grocery store if I would like any assistance with the bags. My self-image says that I do not look like someone that needs this type of assistance! I made the assumption that they looked at me and decided that I actually did need assistance, which I certainly did not. I always would say no with a somewhat indignant tone.

Our second task, after settling in at the Cove, was provisioning for our holiday. After completing the check-out, the usual question was asked, "Would you like some assistance with the bags, sir?" Much to my surprise, I heard myself saying yes! Prior to last year, this would never happen. I found that accepting this change was just fine!

FOOD

The Transformation of the "Dining Out" Experience

One of our favorite activities is eating and when combined with going to a restaurant, it is transformed into an "experience". However, the eating out experience has been forever changed! I have always been "difficult" for the servers in that I would request salad dressing on the side, hold the sauce, could I have a baked potato instead of fries? You get the idea!

The bar has now been raised significantly on this process. I follow my dietary guideline rigorously. They are: no butter, no or very little salt, no fatty foods, nothing deep fried and no egg yolks. Yikes! Gone is a long list of my favorite foods that are now "off limits". Prime rib, barbecued ribs, sauces and gravies and almost all desserts with the exception of a fresh fruit cup – all gone!

I have found that any really good restaurant can accommodate me but care must be taken in giving instructions. Going to a restaurant now is definitely a different experience.

The Challenges of Being a Polite Guest

The challenge of going to a restaurant is a piece of cake when compared to being invited out for dinner to someone's home or to an event like a reception where there is no control over the food. In the latter case, the solution is quite simple: eat anything that "qualifies" and avoid the rest. If this means eating nothing, then so be it. In a crowd, no one is going to notice or care that you are not eating.

Being invited to someone's home is much more complex. The decision here is to what extent do I commit to following my guidelines? What do I do if the entrée is prime rib? What if the host serves linguini already mixed with a cheese cream sauce?

Trying to intervene before the fact is iffy since most people feel that they understand what "healthy eating" is and simply respond, "You'll be fine. There will be lots to eat for you." Unfortunately, in reality this is simply not true. Resolving this dilemma is a work in progress. To date, I have not found an easy solution.

"Wodgy" Breakfasts, Burgers, and Smorgasbords

One of our traditional rituals was to go out on a Saturday or Sunday morning for what I would call a "wodgy breakfast". For a visual on this, all you have to do is tune into Diners, Drive-ins and Dives on the

Food Channel and watch Guy Fieri extol the virtues of local eateries around North America that provide this fare.

Although our weekend indulgences never approached the magnitude of what these diners were serving, I did enjoy ham and eggs and hash brown potatoes along with the odd pancake!

Another "delicacy" I would enjoy on occasion is hamburgers and fries. Guy also does an outstanding job showcasing this American classic. All wodgy fare like barbecued ribs, pot roast and gravy and the like I am sad to say are also definitely off the program for reasons too numerous to mention! The vicarious pleasure of watching Diners and Guy will never be the same!

Finally, I used to look forward to a good smorgasbord, for in the realm of food, we all understand that access to quantity at times can rival or even exceed the importance of quality! Since eating large amounts is no longer a recommended activity for me combined with my lack of control over the food, (you can only eat from the choices that are presented) this periodic dining adventure has also been taken off the program.

Casual Eating Out and Snacking

In some ways, this is one of the biggest differences, because the opportunity for control is almost always absent and the pleasure of being spontaneous is removed. If you want to respect following the guidelines, your choices become quite limited!

You are out and about and get hungry. Stopping for a muffin or scone is not possible since both are usually made from things that are on the "forbidden list". Gone also are treats like a cookie or occasional slice of cake! Similarly, prepared sandwiches fail to qualify. Stopping for a quick burger and fries is also a thing of the past! Restaurants like Subway or Quizno's are great since you can order food exactly the way you want it. However, establishments like these are not always available. In short, no more recreational eating!

See's Candies

Finally, there is one more tasty treat that has suffered the same fate as the "wodgy breakfast". *See's Candies* have been a part of my life for as long as I can remember. A trip to the US was never complete without stopping to pick up a few pounds! After my discharge from the hospital in Honolulu, I was compelled to check the ingredient list when we went to stock up. Much to my disappointment, there were many of my forbidden foods: butter, cream, hydrogenated vegetable oil. See's would no longer be a staple in my repertoire of culinary pleasures. However, one practice that persists is our consumption of dark chocolate with more than 70 percent cocoa mass and no offending additives.

Mandatory Meds

Before January, 2009, I only had one medication that was "legislated", a very low dose of a diuretic to control my blood pressure. Now I am on four medications and a few supplements that have been prescribed by the doctors that I will probably be taking for the rest of my life. I was quite accustomed to taking many pills every day but they were always self-prescribed. There were no consequences in missing a day but now a "miss" is simply not acceptable! Consequently, the discipline of taking my pills at breakfast and at dinner has been institutionalized into my routine. Just one more thing to think about!

Supplements

These changes have already been discussed. I lost my status as a poster boy for the supplementation industry, going from taking more than forty pills a day down to four plus the multivitamin/mineral that was imbedded in my rice protein powder. This change dramatically simplified my life and also saved me thousands of dollars a year! I also must confess that I have not been able to identify any noticeable difference in how I feel after dropping all the supplements. I am left wondering just how much of the information on the value of supplementation is really, "just marketing"!

The Mystery of Losing Weight and Maintaining the Loss is Solved!

I have struggled with losing weight for a long time. My weight when I started teaching at the university in 1969 was around 175 pounds. Over the years, this number gradually crept up and finally settled in the mid to high 190s about twenty years ago where it stuck. Periodically, I would hit 200 and on a few rare occasions would find myself north of 205, but I did not stay there for very long. I never thought of myself as having a weight problem and was certainly not seen that way by others! However, I was always on a mission to drop below 190!

When I went into the hospital in Honolulu I was slightly over 200 pounds and left at around 190. Over the last year, my weight has gradually drifted down and now bounces around the 175 range. I'm back to where I was in 1969! How in the world did I achieve this?

Remember a few of my dietary restrictions: no butter, no high fat foods and one egg yolk a week. If one takes these restrictions seriously, which I have done, then a whole range of potentially fattening foods are immediately taken out of play. Virtually all commercially baked products: cookies, cakes, pastries, donuts, and muffins contain one or more of the offending ingredients, especially egg yolks. Since weight loss is ultimately a function of calories consumed, then removing all these high calorie foods from my diet could not help but have a positive impact on my efforts to lose weight. The nightly practice of snacking on a few cookies is gone and has been replaced by healthier fare. The results speak for themselves.

I also find that I am less interested in consuming really large meals, which has helped as well. Eating properly is discussed in more detail in a later section.

$\mathcal{P}art\,7$

February, 2010 – November, 2013

It's now time to finish the story. Outside of a few notable events described below, the description of these four years is quite brief.

2010

My convalescence proceeded without event this year. However, life has a way of intervening. Towards the end of October, I noticed that I was "bulging" in a place where I previously was not. This prompted a trip to my doctor who calmly reported to me that I had a hernia. I was advised not to lift anything heavy and suspend my pushup regimen, but was cleared to continue exercise walking. An appointment was set with the surgeon for February, 2011 for an assessment and to set a date for my surgery. This seemingly innocent scheduling turned out to have a significant impact on our lives moving forward.

Life reverted to normal with the above adjustments until it was time to secure an extension to our medical travel insurance for our yearly trip to Hawaii. We went to BCAA to make the necessary arrangements and everything seemed in order. The decision was made to come back a few days before our departure to actually pay for the policy. At this time, we had a different agent and what was seen as a non-issue at our first meeting now became a major issue, the pending appointment with the surgeon to deal with my hernia. Any condition that falls in this category is not covered. Ironically, my heart related issues were stable (in medical travel insurance terms) but my hernia was not! This glitch ultimately resulted in us having to cancel our trip to Hawaii in 2010. I simply was not willing to risk travelling and having any hernia-related event not be covered.

In terms of my ongoing convalescence from my operation, everything was proceeding positively.

2011

I met with Dr. Meloche on February 1, who examined me and set the date for my surgery for the afternoon of Wednesday, May 4. It was day surgery, and I would be in the hospital about three to four hours. He reassured me that it was a simple, straightforward procedure. Being an "expert", I was not overly concerned. I was further reassured after learning that Dr. Meloche had a similar record in his specialty performing hernia surgeries as Dr. Grattan had had with his heart surgeries.

The day of my surgery proceeded without event. I drove to the hospital, but Denise drove us home. The experience took me back to when I returned from Hawaii in 2009. I was told not to drive for about a week and to avoid lifting anything heavy. I decided that included my pushups and would refrain from any heavy exercise until I got clearance from the doctor on my follow up visit.

When I attempted to resume my pushup regimen after about nine months, I was absolutely amazed at the dramatic loss of upper body strength that I experienced as a result of my inactivity. I was astonished that my arms were unable to support my body weight! Forget about how many pushups! One pushup was an impossibility. This was the starting point for my pushup regimen. I started with "ladies" pushups (using my knees rather than my toes as the pivot point) and gradually became able to do one pushup. I worked this number up to about fifteen before I decided it was time to switch back to the regular pushup format. I started there at one and when I changed the format of my pushups in the summer of 2013 I had built myself up to eighty. The mantra of this scenario is "Use it or lose it".

I'm delighted to say that my convalescing had really transitioned into a complete return to my previous lifestyle. My medications were stable, and I was feeling fine. My weight was also stable staying within the 172–176 pound range. And thankfully there were no medical travel insurance dramas to interfere with our trip back to Maui in December.

2012

This year was simply a continuation of 2011 minus the drama and recovery from my hernia. My eating regimen continued along with striving to walk 10,000 steps a day and do my pushups. The adjustment to the dietary restrictions was becoming easier to accept and deal with. The year progressed uneventfully from the perspective of my cardiovascular event, and this is a good thing!

We were off to Hawaii again in December without event. However, there were some major disappointments upon our arrival. We were unable to stay at our unit at the Cove because of renovations. We knew this, but we found the alternative accommodations underwhelming. We were much further back from the ocean. The unit was quite dark and the friendly faces at the Cove were absent.

As the line goes "You only know what you've missed when it's gone." Our new "home" on Maui was definitely not the Cove.

2013

This year has proceeded uneventfully with only some minor changes to my overall routine.

Nutrition

If anything, my devotion to my nutritional regimen has strengthened over time. I don't eat any milk fat. This eliminates butter, cheese, whipped cream, and other dairy products except non-fat milk and yogurt. Also, on the recommendation of my cardiologist, I limit myself to one egg yolk per week. This combination of egg yolks and butter effectively eliminates foods such as commercially baked cakes, pies, and pastries, any dessert that is the slightest bit appetizing, many varieties of pasta and a whole range of sauces. Eggs Benedict is definitely off the program; fortunately for me it never was on! Also any fatty cuts of meat such as prime rib are verboten along with processed meats. And finally, deep fried foods, as good as they taste, are also permanently off the program. My only regular "indiscretion" is that I have a little Lite Mayonnaise or Miracle Whip on my sandwiches.

On the positive side I start every day, and by every day I mean 365 days a year, with a protein shake. The recipe is in the Appendix. Another positive outcome is that I have developed all kinds of "healthy treats" that satisfy my sweet tooth, which has not gone away. It's possible to bake very tasty desserts without any of the offending ingredients. Finally, some more good news! Dark chocolate continues to be on the program! And I consume a small amount almost every day. However, I have to admit that I do eat a few cookies after dinner on a semi-regular basis.

Weight

Because of a number of circumstances that were different in our Hawaiian vacation over December/January, we wound up walking much less than we initially planned. The consequence of this was the counter balancing force to account for the consumption of too many cookies was removed so I returned from Hawaii five or so pounds heavier than when I left. My weight has been stable in the 172–175 pound range, but this range had now become 176–179. Yikes! At this writing I am a touch over 176 pounds.

Exercise

In terms of walking, I have been quite conscientious on sticking to my 10,000 steps a day regimen. My target is to meet this goal a minimum of five out of seven days per week. Most days, Denise and I walk for thirty to sixty minutes, rain or shine in Burnaby's Central Park. If I don't reach the requisite 10,000 steps during the day's activities I will make up the balance by walking through the house during commercial breaks of "Diner's Drive Ins and Dives". No one said that you can't look; you just can't touch!

In regards to pushups, I was encouraged to change my regimen from a format where I tried to do as many three-quarter pushups as fast as I can. I was back up to eighty. Then I met Jim Karas who was a Resource to my TEC groups on nutrition and fitness. He recommended that to get full advantage from the pushups, they should be done slowly (to the count of six – three down, three up), and be complete, that is through a full range of motion. Eighty pushups very quickly became ten. Yikes again! My plan continues to be to build the numbers every week, but to date progress beyond fourteen has eluded me.

Medical

I have bi-monthly meetings and a yearly physical with my family physician, Dr. Glanzberg. My blood pressure is monitored regularly and my cholesterol and other "markers" are monitored yearly and any deviations are addressed. Dr. Isserow my cardiologist continues not to be concerned about me in a good way since I did not meet with him this year. My next visit is February, 2014.

Part 8

Why Me? Why This Outcome?

Some Relevant Background

In the early 1980s, I started to get interested in lifestyle issues. This conversion happened haphazardly, without a plan or objective. The major components of this "conversion" are described below with the food-related items listed first followed by exercise and supplementation.

FOOD

"The Truth about Fiber in Your Food"

In 1982, I was on sabbatical from the University of British Columbia and decided to take a road trip to visit my brother who was living in Los Angeles. On the way down, I stopped in Eugene to visit the University of Oregon where I did my graduate work. While wandering through the campus, I noticed that there was a book sale at the library. So not being able to pass up a potential bargain, I went in. There was a large table strewn with books that were on sale right by the door. I started rummaging through them and *The Truth About Fiber in Your Food* by Lawrence Galton caught my eye.

The book was all about transit times, cancer rates, and their relationship to the amount of fiber consumed. The typical diet in Africa fared much better than the one in North America in terms of fiber consumption. I bought the book and made the decision consciously to add fiber to my daily regime.

This event marked the beginning of my eccentric eating habits and opened me to no end of ridicule and derision in the years to come. I bought a small, zippered leather pouch into which I put wheat bran. I always had my pouch with me and whenever soup was served, I added a tablespoon of bran. I also received a gift of a beautiful lacquered box with the quote below in which to store my bran.

"Man who eat plenty of fiber feel bran new."

Healthy Eating

Following my conversion to wheat bran, I also began generally to watch what I ate. This involved being conscious of fat content and cutting down on "fast foods" and deep fried foods. I stopped using butter on my bread, generally avoided processed meats and eliminated rich sauces, which I did not care for much anyway. In addition, I started to become aware of my consumption of sugar and white flour, which resulted in a reduction of cakes, cookies, pastries, and soft drinks in my diet.

As this process evolved, I also became increasingly interested in cooking and baking "healthy" alternatives to the standard dishes.

Another practice that I adopted was starting my day with a protein shake. I was doing this a long time before it became popular.

I have been a TEC Chair since 1987. The Executive Committee (TEC – Renamed Vistage in the United States) is a professional development organization for CEOs, presidents and key executives in organizations. Groups of 10–16 meet monthly for a full day, half of which is devoted to hearing a speaker on a topic of interest to the group and the balance of the day is spent with the members brainstorming solutions to each other's challenges.

It was in this capacity that I met Joe Dillon in April of 1999. His topic was Producing Peak Performance. Joe introduced me to the practice. I found that having a shake in the morning solved a number of "problems" simultaneously.

It removed the question, "What am I going to have for breakfast this morning?" for these reasons:

It was a balanced, nutritious meal.

It was quick.

It removed all cravings for the "bad" breakfast foods such as muffins, Danish pastries, donuts and breakfast sandwiches served up at fast food restaurants.

EXERCISE

"Power Walking in the Park"

I've never liked jogging, but I have always appreciated the importance of being physically active. In the mid-1980s, I discovered power walking, and this activity seemed to be the best of both worlds. It provided an aerobic workout and avoided having to jog!

Living in Vancouver, we have a wonderful, world famous resource called the Seawall Path in Stanley Park. I would make it a habit to walk at least once or twice a week there accompanied by my cousin, who would jog while I walked, or by another friend whom I converted into being a devotee of power walking.

I walked an 8-kilometer course (5 miles) on the Seawall. My target was to complete the five miles in under sixty minutes. This pace was fast enough not only to get an excellent aerobic workout but also sufficient to pass a significant percentage of the female joggers, something that many of them found quite irritating but delighted me! My best time was 52.5 minutes, which was 10.5-minute miles. This pace was certainly not fast enough to break any world records, but it was definitely a great day. (The Olympic race walking pace is below 6-minute miles!) Since then, walking almost daily has been a part of my routine, albeit, not at my record pace.

"Heavy Hands"

Joe also introduced us to the practice of working out with light hand weights. The procedure was simple and the results, impressive. By walking for thirty minutes with a few pounds in each hand doing a variety of movements, you not only get an aerobic workout, but also build muscle tone and endurance. I have continued this activity intermittently until I started to visit a chiropractor, who recommended that I not use the hand weights while walking since they might aggravate my neck.

SUPPLEMENTATION

In Search of a Healthier Lifestyle through the Wonders of "Science"

Adding vitamins, minerals and other micronutrients to our diet has become very popular. There are four basic approaches to the practice:

1. Eating a balanced diet will provide everything that we need.
2. Depleted soils no longer produce foods that contain the required nutrients so supplementation is necessary.
3. Adding additional vitamins and minerals is beneficial, regardless of our diet.
4. The isolated nutrients will never be able to provide the same value as consuming the whole foods that originally contained them.
   - Regardless, the consumption of supplements is thriving!

A Personal Case Study

I have until quite recently been a supporter of taking vitamin and mineral supplements to enhance quality of life. As mentioned, I used to take around forty supplements a day believing that the only negative consequence would be "expensive urine" but after my "event", I have had my initial practice dramatically altered to the point where I now consume very few.

Part 9

———

Suggestions for Improving Your Overall Cardiovascular Health

Based on my background provided in the preceding section and my experiences since my procedure in January 2009, the following suggestions are offered based on the risk assessment guide that was introduced at the beginning of this book.

The dilemma in this section of the book is to find the right balance between generalities that provide very little useful information on the one hand, and the enormous amount of existing knowledge in each of these categories on the other. We are like Goldilocks looking for the bowl of porridge that's "just right". The approach that has been adopted is to provide lists of actionable points under each category.

Medical and Dental Health, Medical Markers, and Heredity or Genetic Predisposition

The point here is to be aware of the importance of these three categories and to ensure that they are not neglected in your quest for cardiovascular health.

Action Points for your Consideration:

- Get a doctor if you don't have one.
- Have regular medical checkups.
- Know and monitor your blood pressure.
- Know and monitor your cholesterol numbers.
- Know and monitor blood sugar and any other tests that your doctor believes are important.
- Know and monitor your weight and take action when it goes above a healthy range.
- Get a dentist if you don't have one.
- Have regular dental checkups and visits to the dental hygienist.
- Be aware of your family history; your diligence should increase with the frequency of close family and relatives who suffered from or have cardiovascular disease.

Nutritional Habits

Nutrition is the most important factor over which you have direct control to affect your cardiovascular health.

Action Points for your Consideration:

Strive to eat foods in their natural rather than processed form. (i.e., an apple is preferable to apple juice, a potato is better than potato chips.)

Make fruits, vegetables, and to a lesser extent, grains, seeds, and nuts the major component of your diet. Remember that many of these foods are non-animal sources of protein.

Protein from animal sources falls on a continuum from most desirable to least desirable: The continuum ranges from fish to poultry to lean forms of red meat (beef [preferably grass fed], pork, lamb, etc.) to processed meats (ham, sausages, salami, hot dogs, and bologna, etc.)

If choosing protein from animal sources, select those that are lower in fat. (i.e., extra lean ground beef is preferable to regular ground beef.)

Limit your consumption of saturated fats and ensure that you consume sufficient quantities of omega 3, 6, and 9 oils.

Avoid the consumption of hydrogenated fats and avoid or limit any food that is deep fried.

Limit your consumption of sugar and other refined carbohydrates. (e.g., cakes, cookies, pastries, donuts, and other commercially baked goods.)

When choosing dairy products, select low fat or non-fat varieties (skim milk, nonfat yogurt and cottage cheese, etc.)

Limit or avoid cheese. It's a high fat food! (Yes, this means pizza.)

Limit or avoid the consumption of "the five basic non-food groups". These are: sugar, salt, fat, white flour, and alcohol.

Eat consciously. Limit and monitor your intake of calories, sodium, fat, sugar, refined carbohydrates, alcohol, and caffeine.

Ensure that your diet includes a sufficient amount of soluble and insoluble fiber.

Be aware that most meals occur in a social context. Do not let this context persuade you to make bad choices.

There's a vast amount of information available on nutrition. The strategy here is to apply Pareto's Principle. It's not necessary to get caught up in the detail or fine points; 80 percent of your positive outcomes will come from 20 percent of the information. The points above are a summary of this 20 percent. For a more detailed explanation of these guidelines refer to my book: *Nutritional Intelligence: Eating for Life on the 80/20 Plan* (nutritionalintelligence.com)

Exercise Habits

As a general principle, the more we keep moving the better. With this in mind, there are three primary objectives to be achieved from exercising: Aerobic capacity, strength, and flexibility.

Aerobic Capacity

This category includes jogging, cycling, swimming, brisk walking, and any other activity that raises your heart rate. It is an essential piece in any exercise regimen. There are many levels at which one can be engaged ranging from the recreational walker or cyclist to the marathon runner.

There is more information available than you would ever need to know about jogging, running, cycling, etc. It's well beyond the scope of this book to get into any of it.

Strength

Strength training is any physical exercise focusing on the use of resistance to build muscle capacity and endurance. There are a wide variety of approaches to achieve this ranging from free weights to machines; to entire programs like CrossFit.

Maintaining strength and muscle mass as we age becomes increasingly important since they are the crucial ingredients in maintaining stamina, preventing falls and mitigating injury if we do fall. Everyone needs to be actively engaged in maintaining their strength as they age. Not debatable! The good news here is that you can start anytime. People well into their eighties and nineties have been able to increase their strength simply by exercising with soup cans!

Flexibility

Maintaining a range of motion in all parts of our body is important as we age. There are also a wide variety of approaches to achieve flexibility ranging from different types of yoga, Pilates, and a wide variety of stretching exercises.

Action Points for your Consideration:

Have some form of aerobic activity embedded in your day. If this is not possible, settle for three or four times a week.

Buy a pedometer and track your number of steps per day. Aiming for 10,000 steps at least five days a week is a reasonable target.

Find a strength training regimen that is best suited to your personal situation and lifestyle and then follow through on it. The question is not whether you should do this but how you're going to do it.

There are many choices for enhancing flexibility. Find an option that suits your lifestyle and then consistently practice it.

Personality and Mental Factors

Our state of mind has a significant role to play in our cardiovascular health. Below are some steps that you can take to enhance your health in this arena.

Personality Type and State of Mind
Action Points for your Consideration:

Know whether you are a "Type A" or "Type B" personality and be aware that defaulting automatically to "Type A" behaviors such as impatience and anger can have a negative impact on your cardiovascular health.

Having positive expectations about outcomes is also more conducive to cardiovascular health. Habitual worrying about undesirable outcomes can have a negative impact on your health over time.

Lifestyle Stress

There are a number of healthy habits that can be adopted to combat the normal stress that is generated in our daily lives. Below is a list from which you can pick and choose:

Action Points for your Consideration:

Get seven to eight hours of sleep every night. This practice gives your body an opportunity to rejuvenate and sets you up to perform optimally the next day. Prolonged sleep deprivation can have serious health consequences. The practice of sleeping four to five hours a night is not sustainable over time.

Include meditation, spend quiet and/or contemplative time, relax or become engaged in any activity that takes you "away" from your daily stresses as a regular part of your daily routine.

Nurture and develop a social support network that you can rely on when you need it.

Take action to deal with unproductive, dysfunctional, or toxic relationships in your work or home environment.

Consciously manage your time so as to avoid last minute "pressures" and demands.

Unhealthy "Bad" Habits

If you possess any of the "bad" habits, you will be much better off without them. Do whatever you need to do to take the necessary action. Get a buddy, find a support group, start a program. Take action!

Action Points for your Consideration:

- Don't smoke. And if you do smoke, quit now!
- Limit your consumption of alcohol. If you don't drink, don't start.
- Remove fast food from your diet.
- If you have a sedentary lifestyle, abandon it, and get active.

Part 10

Some Concluding Thoughts

Being a "Real Man" Might Just Kill You! And it Doesn't Matter if You are a Man or a Woman!

Real men don't complain. Real men push through the discomfort or pain. Real men are "indestructible"! Being a "real man" might not be very good for you. One of the things that I learned through this adventure was that heart disease can manifest itself in many forms, many of which are quite subtle. Everyone should become familiar with the subtle signs that there might be trouble, things like indigestion or a sense of just not feeling quite right. I had been experiencing uneasy sensations, which I referred to as "spells" for quite a few years, but I never connected the dots. These episodes would appear infrequently, once every six months to a year or so, and would pass within a few hours. The symptoms were vague and difficult to describe. In retrospect, I suspect it was coronary artery disease but none of the tests that I took, and there were many, showed anything.

My suggestion – Be a "hypochondriac"! It's better to err on the side of over diligence.

Have Someone "In Your Corner" Who Loves You and Will Care for You

If left to my own devices, I would not have gone to the clinic on Thursday morning without Denise's insistence. Would the ultimate outcome have been different if I had not gone? Who knows! But given the extent of my blockages, there is a good chance that I would have had an "event" resulting in heart damage prior to getting to a hospital or worse. In these matters, it's much better to be too soon rather than a bit late!

Do you have someone in your life who is concerned about and monitors your health? When we were growing up our mothers typically played this role. It's not a bad idea to ensure that we always have someone close to us that is "watching our back" in this regard.

Taking Care of Yourself Takes Priority Over Everything Else

Another bit of good fortune that was factored into my experience was being on holiday. There were no intruding agendas or demands. I often think about what would have happened if I had been at home. It's much harder to cancel and/or reschedule work commitments in order to accommodate an unplanned visit to the doctor.

Since my symptoms were ambiguous, I could always justify "pushing through". I always would feel better in a while and would resume my regular routine. I never had the experience where I had to leave a commitment because I was not feeling well.

Remember, your health is more important than anything else. Don't get your priorities confused. Take care of yourself first. Everything else can wait, even if you believe it cannot!

Epilogue

May 3, 2019

As I stated in the Foreword, writing the book was significantly delayed for a variety of reasons. So now we find ourselves just over three months beyond ten years after "the event". An advantage of the delay is that what has happened to me is not theory, projection/ conjecture nor "hope" but fact.

How has my life changed? There are many responses to this question. In no particular order they are:

WEIGHT

When I was admitted to Straub, I weighed between 200 and 205 pounds. Now my weight falls in the range between 157 and 162 pounds. I am around fifty pounds lighter now! It is important to note that I have never tried to lose weight, but I have significantly changed many aspects of my behavior.

DIET

Beginning with diet, Dr. Isserow gave me two direct orders: no more butter and one egg yolk a week. I took him beyond literally. I chose to avoid all forms of milk fat, which along with butter includes, cheese and all dairy that is not fat free. I have held fast to this rule since 2009. One result is I have become the master of the cheeseless pizza!

I also eat only one egg yolk a week. However, I do cheat a bit on this in that I have lite mayonnaise on my sandwiches. However, what this guideline combined with the avoidance of milk fat achieves is the complete removal of almost all commercially baked products from my diet: cookies, cakes, pastries, donuts, muffins, etc. It is important to note that I have not lost my "sweet tooth" but now I bake all my treats so that they conform to my guidelines, which is not a problem. Skim milk, egg whites and nut/seed oils are all workable substitutes for the forbidden ingredients.

I also generally avoid all deep fried foods, high fat cuts of meat (beef prime rib and pork ribs, etc.), and processed meats such as salamis and bologna. It's important to note that prior to 2009, beef prime rib and pork ribs were viewed as "treats" which definitely were not avoided!

Eating in restaurants can be a challenge but good restaurants are usually able to accommodate me. To get the picture, just imagine me minus the "abuse" as Jack Nicholson's character in *"Five Easy Pieces" trying to order toast!*

EXERCISE

I have been consistent in walking 10,000 steps most days. In 2018 I walked 86 days beyond my target of 10,000 steps, five out of every seven days. I recently have had a "flu bug" that sidelined my push-up program but when I stopped in February, I was doing 76 push-ups in three sets three to four times a week. I also have been doing other weight bearing exercises but on a less regular basis. Finally, my stretching routine has suffered a bit in terms of consistency!

PROFESSSIONAL ACTIVITY

I continue to chair three Key Executive Groups for TEC Canada (The Executive Committee/Vistage) and consult to organizations on strategic planning initiatives.

Appendices

A. Steve's Nutritionally Intelligent Protein Shake

What follows is probably more than you want to know about making a protein shake but I thought I would give you everything and you can "pick and choose". There are many ways to do this. What is provided here is my current "version."

Equipment Required

Blender (6-cup plus capacity) and Coffee Grinder (preferably one that is used solely for this purpose).

Ingredients Required

- Fruit (fresh or frozen): bananas, pears, plums, blueberries, raspberries, strawberries, peaches, cherries, mangos, melons, papayas, etc.
- Leafy Greens: spinach, black kale, etc.
- Raw Unsalted Nuts: almonds, walnuts, etc. (I use 12 almonds and the equivalent of about 28 grams/1 ounce of walnuts.)

- Seeds - flax, pumpkin and sunflower ($1\frac{1}{2}$ heaping teaspoons of each) and Grains – oat bran, wheat bran and psyllium fiber ($1\frac{1}{2}$ heaping tablespoons of each), etc.
- Spices, etc.: Cinnamon and turmeric (Turmeric is purported to have multiple health benefits as does the cinnamon and the cinnamon masks the taste of the turmeric ($\frac{1}{4}$ teaspoon of each), raw green tea (I use organic Gunpowder – $1\frac{1}{2}$ teaspoons. Note: This is a variety of green tea!).
- Protein Powder: 90% whey, soy, rice, or other varieties of vegetable-based protein. (I currently use a heaping scoop of a rice/pea protein based product called MediClear® from Thorne Research along with a scoop of Amino Complex and Magnesium Bisglycinate both from Thorne Research [using the scoops provided].)
- Liquid – $3\frac{1}{2}$–4 cups of water. (You could also use skim milk, nut milk, rice milk or soy milk. I would avoid fruit juices simply because of their high sugar content. Your choice.)

Directions

Since there is some preparation required, I recommend that you prepare the dry ingredients for a number of breakfasts at the same time. I prepare about two weeks at a time. Grind the seeds, grains and green tea in the coffee grinder and place the powder into a plastic sandwich bag. Add the nuts, protein powder, turmeric, cinnamon, Amino Complex and Magnesium Bisglycinate to each bag. Store the bags in the refrigerator.

1. Put about 1–3 cups of a variety of fresh and/or frozen fruit into the blender. Use bananas if you are not concerned about sugar content. They give the shake a nice consistency. (Use as

much or as little fruit according to your taste. If you use more fruit, your shake will have a thicker consistency.) [Currently I use one banana, some honeydew melon, papaya, 10–15 raspberries, ½ cup of blueberries, ½ an avocado and ½ a Blood or Cara orange. This will vary depending on what is available.]

2. Finely chop the kale and place it in the blender [I use the equivalent of one large leaf.]
3. Empty a bag of the dry ingredients into the blender.
4. Pour the water (or your choice of liquid) into the blender. Blend and drink! ENJOY! I find that the shake takes care of my needs for food until the early afternoon, and if I have it later in the morning, I am usually good until dinner! Another advantage of the shake is that it provides you with way more than your daily requirement of fiber.

B. Steve's Nutritionally Intelligent Pancakes

(FOR THE PURIST)

Equipment Required

Coffee Grinder (preferably one that is not used for grinding coffee!) and a whisk

Ingredients

- ⅓ cup of flax seeds
- ⅓ cup of oat bran

- ⅓ cup of buckwheat
- ⅓ cup of wheat bran
- 1 heaping tablespoon of raw pumpkin seeds
- 1 heaping tablespoon of raw sesame seeds
- 1 heaping tablespoon of raw sunflower seeds
- 1 to 2 teaspoons of baking powder
- 2 eggs or 4 egg whites*
- 1½ to 2 cups of skim milk*
- 1 tablespoon of oil – I use organic safflower oil
- A wide variety of fruit may also be added to the pancakes if you wish

NOTE: Do not use psyllium. It absorbs too much liquid and will turn the batter into the consistency of a thick mud!

Directions

- Mix all the seeds, oat bran, flax, wheat bran, and buckwheat together.
- Grind them in batches in the coffee grinder until they are a fine powder.
- In a large mixing bowl, combine the ground material with the baking powder and mix well.
- Reserve a tablespoon or two for coating any fruit that you might be adding.
- Put a cup of the milk in a bowl and add the eggs or egg whites and the oil and whisk until blended.
- Add the milk/egg/oil mixture to the dry ingredients and mix well.
- Then gradually add the additional milk until the batter reaches the desired consistency. (You might have to add more

milk while you are making the pancakes since the batter will thicken as it sits.)

- Add the fruit. (Optional)
- Fry on a lightly oiled skillet and cook like you would a regular pancake.

Additional Thoughts

- You might find that you need less baking powder.
- If you are not sensitive to gluten, you can add wheat berries as one of the ingredients to be ground.
- The recipe is quite flexible. Experiment with different ingredients and different proportions until you settle on a favorite.
- One advantage of this recipe is that it can be adapted to accommodate a gluten free diet simply through the choice of ingredients.
- It enables the nutritionally minded to have healthy pancakes that do not contain any highly refined carbohydrates.
- * If you wish to avoid animal protein, omit the eggs and substitute soy, rice or almond milk for the skim milk and increase the baking powder from 1–2 teaspoons to 1–2 tablespoons.

ENJOY!

Steve's Nutritionally Intelligent Pancakes (for the Expedient Minimalist)

Equipment Required

- A whisk

Ingredients

- 1 ½ cups of Bob's Red Mill Organic Whole Wheat Flour
- ½ cup of oat bran
- ½ cup of wheat bran
- 2 to 3 teaspoons of baking powder
- 1 egg or 2 egg whites*
- 1 to 2 cups of skim milk*
- 2 tablespoon of oil – I use organic safflower oil
- A wide variety of fruit may also be added to the pancakes if you wish

Directions

- In a large mixing bowl, combine the flour, oat bran and wheat bran with the baking powder and mix well.
- Reserve a tablespoon or two for coating any fruit that you might be adding.
- Put a cup of the milk in a bowl and add the egg or egg whites and the oil and whisk until blended.
- Add the milk/egg/oil mixture to the dry ingredients and mix well.

- Then gradually add the additional milk until the batter reaches the desired consistency. (You might have to add more milk while you are making the pancakes since the batter will thicken as it sits.)
- Add the fruit. (Optional)
- Fry on a lightly oiled skillet and cook like you would a regular pancake.

Additional Thoughts

- You might find that you need less baking powder.
- The recipe is quite flexible. Experiment with different ingredients and different proportions until you settle on a favorite.
- One advantage of this recipe is that it can be adapted to accommodate a gluten free diet simply through the choice of ingredients.
- It enables the nutritionally minded to have healthy pancakes that do not contain any highly refined carbohydrates.
- * If you wish to avoid animal protein, omit the eggs and substitute soy, rice or almond milk for the skim milk and increase the baking powder from 2–3 teaspoons to 1–2 tablespoons.

ENJOY!

C. Supplements

PRE "EVENT" VITAMIN LIST

These are the supplements that I took on a regular basis prior to January 8, 2009.

The pills are listed somewhat alphabetically (except the multivitamin) with the brand name or manufacturer identified by the superscripted number.

- Multivitamin (The Legend for Men – Max Stress/Activity[1]):
- Beta Carotene
- Vitamin A
- Vitamin D3
- Vitamin E
- Vitamin C
- Vitamin B1
- Vitamin B2
- Vitamin B6
- Vitamin B12
- Niacinamide
- Folic Acid
- Biotin
- Pantothenic Acid
- Calcium
- Magnesium
- Zinc
- Iodine
- Manganese
- Potassium
- Chromium

- Selenium
- Molybdenum
- Vanadium
- Choline Citrate
- Inositol
- Methionine

Additional Supplements

- Alpha-Lipoic Acid[12] 250 mg
- Anti-Oxidant Supreme[9] 300 mg (Pine Bark and Grape Seed Extracts)
- Ascorbyl Palmitate[5] 500 mg
- BetaCareAll[7] (Mixed Carotenoid Complex) 25,000 IU
- Calcium Supplement
- Cal-Mag Supreme[9] 500 mg (Calcium, Magnesium, Potassium, Strontium, Boron, Vitamin D)
- Chromium Picolinate[5] 200 mcg
- CoEnzyme Q10[7] 60 mg
- Copper Sebacate[11] 4 mg
- Cranberry Extract[9] 800 mg
- EPA/DHA[3] 360 mg/240 mg
- Ester-C Supreme[8] 500 mg
- Folic Acid[9] 800 mcg. (+ Vitamin B12)
- Gamma E[2] (Vitamin E) 200 IU
- Glucosamine & Chondroitin Sulfates[13] 900 mg
- [Glutathione] Reduced Glutathione[13] 500 mg
- Grapefruit Pectin[5] 1,000 mg
- N'Acetyl L-Cysteine[7] 500 mg
- NutraView[6] (Lutein, Zinc, Vitamin C, Blueberry, Bilberry)
- Optizinc[9] 30 mg

- Provex CV[6] (Grape Skin and Seed Extract, Proteases, Ginkgo Biloba, Bilberry, Quercetin)
- Red Yeast Rice[4] 600 mg
- Red Reishi Mushroom[20, 12]
- Replenex[6] (Calcium, Glucosamine HCl, Ginger Root, Bromelain, Green Tea Extract)
- Rutin[7] 250 mg
- Saw Palmetto[10] 160 mg
- Selenium [7] 50 mcg
- Ultra Prim Primrose Oil[7] 500 mg

I also added a number of supplements to my protein shake then, which I took six mornings a week. Following are the products that I put in the shake along with some fruit, usually a banana and some blueberries or strawberries and 2.5 cups of water. (Currently, I do not add any of them!)

- Antioxidant EFA Oil Blend[16]
- Card-D-Ribose[12]
- [Vitamin D in liquid form] Bio-D-Mulsion[14]
- Maca Root (Maca Sure) [16]
- Magnesium Citrate[12]
- Microhydrin[18]
- MSM Powder[9]
- Tea [Green] Matcha Tea[15]
- Tea [White][15]
- Tea [Rooibos][15]
- Trace Minerals {in liquid form} (Foundation of Life) [9]
- Udo's 3-6-9 Oil Blend[17]
- Vega Whole Food Smoothie Infusion[16]
- Whey Protein Isolate - 90[19]

Brand KEY:

1. Nu Life
2. Enerex
3. Alive and Well Natural Health Therapies
4. Solaray
5. Source Naturals
6. Melaleuca
7. Natural Factors
8. Sisu
9. Nutra Research International
10. Herbal Factors
11. Allergy Research Group
12. Finlandia
13. AOR
14. Biotics Research Corp.
15. AIYA Tea Company (Muzi)
16. Sequel Naturals Ltd.
17. Flora
18. USA Royal Body Care Inc.
19. Vitalus Nutrition
20. Nikkei

POST "EVENT" VITAMIN LIST

These are the supplements that I currently take on a regular basis subsequent to my encounters with the doctors in Hawaii and Dr. Ryder in Vancouver.

(Note: This list of contents of MediClear are from the 2009 - 2010 version of the product. However, the contents of the current

version are, with few exceptions/changes, the same. This information is offered as an example of the wide range of vitamin/minerals
that the product contains.)

- MediClear Rice/Pea Protein (Thorne Research – www.thorne.
  com) See the list below for the contents.
- Rice Protein 6.25 g
- Pea Protein 6.25 g
- Glycine 825 mg
- Medium Chain Triglycerides 750 mg
- ((Palm Oil / Coconut Oil) Elaeis guineensis /Cocos nucifera))
- L-Glutamine 250 mg
- L-Lysine 250 mg
- Calcium (Calcium Citrate) 150 mg
- Vitamin C (Ascorbic Acid) 150 mg
- Quercetin (Dimorphandra mollis) (seed) 125 mg
- Magnesium (Magnesium Citrate) 75 mg
- Taurine 55 mg
- Methyl Sulfonyl Methane (MSM) 50 mg
- Potassium (Potassium Citrate) 50 mg
- Betaine (Trimethylglycine) 25 mg
- N-Acetyl-L-Cysteine 25 mg
- Pantothenic Acid (Calcium-D-Pantothenate) 25 mg
- Vitamin E (d-Alpha Tocopherol) (25 IU) 16.8 mg ATE*
- Choline Citrate (Choline Dihydrogen Citrate) 15 mg
- Vitamin B3 (Niacinamide) 15 mg
- Green Tea extract (leaf) (Camellia sinensis) 25 mg
- L-Glutathione 12.5 mg
- Vitamin B1 (Thiamin Hydrochloride) 6 mg
- Vitamin B6 (Pyridoxal 5'-Phosphate) 5 mg
- Zinc (Zinc Picolinate) 5 mg
- Vitamin B3 (Niacin) 4 mg

- Vitamin B2 (Riboflavin 5'-Phosphate Sodium) 2.5 mg
- Beta Carotene (from Mixed Carotenes) (1,500 IU) 900 mcg
- Manganese (Manganese Citrate) 750 mcg
- Vitamin A (Palmitate) (1,000 IU) 302 mcg RAE**
- Folate (5-Methyltetrahydrofolate) 150 mcg
- Biotin 75 mcg
- Boron (Boron Citrate) 50 mcg
- Chromium (Chromium (III) Picolinate) 50 mcg
- Selenium (L-Selenomethionine) 35 mcg
- Molybdenum (Molybdenum Citrate) 25 mcg
- Vanadium (Vanadium Citrate) 25 mcg
- Vitamin B12 (Methylcobalamin) 25 mcg
- Vitamin D3 (Cholecalciferol) (200 IU) 5 mcg

The list below are the supplements that I take separately:
- Amino Complex (Thorne Research) (Powder added to shake packet)
- Magnesium Bisglycinate (Thorne Research) (Powder added to shake packet)
- Magnesium Citramate (Thorne Research) 135 mg
- Cysteplus [N-Acetyl-Cysteine] (Thorne Research) 500 mg
- Vitamin D3 (Thorne Research)
- Fish Oil Concentrate (Selekta – A. N. Tyler Professional Formulation) 1000 mg - EPA 300 mg, DHA 200mg
- Super Saw Palmetto (PhytoPharmica) 160 mg

D. Non-Prescription Remedies and Supplements (G. B. Ryder, M.D.)

All medications and supplements (whether prescription drugs, herbal remedies, vitamin or mineral supplements, essential oils, homeopathics, etc.) must obey the same pharmacological principles. All pharmacologically-active ingredients have three possible effects: positive, neutral, or negative. These three possible effects vary with each individual and also vary with dosage. Secondly, even when you are taking the correct medication, you must take it at the right dosage (for you as an individual) and for a sufficient period of time to achieve any benefit.

A significant number of people also react to the "non-active ingredients" in tablets, gels, and liquids such as binders, fillers, excipients, coloring agents, flavoring agents, etc.

There are currently no regulations in North America (nor Asia) regarding the production, packaging, marketing, advertising claims, purity, safety, effectiveness, standardization, nor even the contents of over 50,000 non-prescription products available locally. As a result, there is often considerable variation in the same pharmacologically-active substance from one brand to another. Without quality control, there can even be significant variation between batches of the same medication/supplement from the same manufacturer. Many investigations have shown that there are often considerable discrepancies between what is written on the label and what is actually in the bottle. Unfortunately, there are very few brands of remedies/supplements in North America that are pharmaceutical-grade and standardized. (Beware all the misleading advertising and unsubstantiated claims – we live in a world of free speech, but you must separate fact from fiction – advertising versus scientific proof). In contrast, government regulations in Germany ensure effectiveness, safety, standardization and pharmaceutical-grade ingredients in all herbal and homeo-pathic remedies.

Adverse reactions to medications and supplements (or their "non-active ingredients") not only harm you (and waste your money), but these toxic reactions often block the beneficial effects of some of your other medications and supplements. Since every one of us is geneti-cally different, we respond (or react) differently to all medications (both prescription and non-prescription). Only a fully qualified pro-fessional can hope to help you individualize your treatment program. In order to optimize benefits and minimize adverse reactions, one must use the least number of beneficial remedies and supplements, use only pharmaceutical-grade ingredients with standardized dosage, and minimize "non-active ingredients".

Conclusion

Now I take five supplements in pill form, two in powder form and the multivitamin mineral in my shake. Then I took twenty-nine supple-ments in pill form including the multivitamin plus ten or more addi-tions to my shake at various times.

I have not noticed any difference in my overall health with the reduction in my consumption of the supplements. They certainly did not prevent my "event" but it's hard to determine whether or not they played any role in mitigating the severity of what I experienced.

The allure of finding a quick fix or a shortcut to greater health is quite compelling so the supplement industry continues to thrive. The quest for the "magic bullet" is alive and well!

Bibliography

(Author's Note: These references deal with nutrition and diet. References related to cardiovascular health and disease are available from your cardiologist, family physician and the internet.)

- Campbell, T. Colin and Campbell, Thomas M. *The China Study: Startling Implications for Diet, Weight Loss and Long Term Health.* Dallas: BenBella Books Inc., 2006.
- Cassels, Alan. "Diabetes Wars: Bad Choices Are Costly." *The Vancouver Sun*, March 4, 2011, A13.
- Crawford, Tiffany. "Check the Label: What You Find May Surprise You." *The Vancouver Sun*, Wednesday, March 16, 2011, A11.
- Crawford, Tiffany. "Juiced: Sugar in a Bottle." *The Vancouver Sun*, Wednesday, March 16, 2011, A8.
- Esselstyn Jr., Caldwell B. *Prevent and Reverse Heart Disease.* New York: Avery, 2007.
- Fayerman, Pamela. "A Weighty Issue: How Much Sugar is Too Much?" *The Vancouver Sun*, Tuesday, March 15, 2011, A6.
- Fuhrman, Joel. *Eat to Live: The Amazing Nutrient-Rich Program For Fast and Sustained Weight Loss*, Revised Edition. New York: Little, Brown and Company, 2001.
- Galton, Lawrence. *The Truth about Fiber in Your Food.* New York: Crown Publishers, Inc., 1976.
- Goleman, Daniel. *Emotional Intelligence: Why It Can Matter More Than IQ.* New York: Bantam Books, 1996.
- Kurzwell, Raymond. *The 10% Solution for A Healthy Life.* New York: Crown Publishers, Inc., 1993.
- Kushi, Michio with Jack, Alex. *The Cancer Prevention Diet.* New York: St. Martin's Press, 1993.

- Marks, Stephen. *Nutritional Intelligence®: Eating for Life on the 80/20 Plan*. (Second Edition), 2017.
- Ornish, Dean. *Eat More, Weigh Less*. New York: HarperCollins, Publishers, Inc., 1993.
- Pennington, Jean A. T. and Church, Helen Nichols. *Bowes and Church's Food Values of Portions Commonly Used*. Philadelphia: J.B. Lippincott Company, 1985.
- Roizen, Michael F. and Oz, Mehmet C. *You, The Owner's Manual*. New York: HarperCollins Publishers, Inc., 2005.
- ——*You, on a Diet*. New York: Simon & Schuster, Inc., 2006.
- ——*You, Staying Young*. New York: Simon & Schuster, Inc., 2007.
- Schmidt, Sarah. "Food Labels Often Untrue, Government Tests Find." *The Vancouver Sun, Friday*, September 3, 2010, B3.
- —— "Inaccurate Claims on Packaging 'Everywhere.'" *The Vancouver Sun*, Tuesday, March 8 2011, B1.
- Stainsby, Mia. "Sweet Without Sugar." *The Vancouver Sun*, Tuesday, March 15, 2011, A6.
- Vancouver Sun Editorial: "Taking Control of the Sugar in Our Food, Drinks." *The Vancouver Sun*, Friday, March 18, 2011, A12.
- Thompson, Rob, *The Glycemic Load Diet*. New York: McGraw-Hill, 2006.

Newsletters

- *Nutrition Action Health Letter*. Jacobson, Michael, Ed. Toronto: Center for Science in the Public Interest.
- The University of California, *Berkeley Wellness Letter*. Swartzberg, John, Ed. New York: University Health Publishing.

Web Sites

- Centers for Disease Control and Prevention (http://www.cdc. gov/)
- Continuum Partners – Dietary Fiber http://www.wehealny. org/healthinfo/dietaryfiber/fibercontentchart.html)
- Health Canada – Smoking and Nicotine (http://www.hc-sc. gc.ca/hc-ps/tobac-tabac/body-corps/addiction-dependance-eng.php

Contacting the Authors

Denise and Steve are available to talk about their experiences dealing with cardio-vascular disease focusing on lifestyle and nutrition to interested groups or organizations.

In addition, Steve is available to conduct workshops on the above topics for groups that are interested in engaging in the topic in a more interactive format.

The authors can be contacted at: sl@stephenmarks.com

www.ingramcontent.com/pod-product-compliance
Lightning Source LLC
Chambersburg PA
CBHW020517290526
45786CB00002B/645